REGIONAL ANATOMY COLOURING BOOK

I. Lennox MMAA
Senior Medical Artist, Department of Medical Illustration,
University of Edinburgh, Edinburgh

F. Kristmundsdottir BSc PhD
Lecturer, Department of Anatomy,
University of Edinburgh, Edinburgh

J. Shaw BDS PhD FDS RCSEd
Head of Department, Department of Anatomy,
University of Edinburgh, Edinburgh

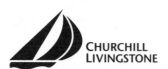

CHURCHILL
LIVINGSTONE

NEW YORK EDINBURGH LONDON MADRID MELBOURNE SAN FRANCISCO AND TOKYO 1997

CHURCHILL LIVINGSTONE
Medical Division of Pearson Professional Limited

Distributed in the United States of America by Churchill
Livingstone Inc., 650 Avenue of the Americas, New York, N.Y.
10011, and by associated companies, branches and representatives
throughout the world.

First published 1997

ISBN 0 443 05727 3

British Library Cataloguing in Publication Data
A catalogue record for this book is available from the British
Library.

Library of Congress Cataloging in Publication Data
A catalog record for this book is available from the Library of
Congress.

Medical knowledge is constantly changing. As new information
becomes available, changes in treatment, procedures, equipment
and the use of drugs become necessary. The authors and the
publishers have, as far as it is possible, taken care to ensure that
the information given in this text is accurate and up to date.
However, readers are strongly advised to confirm that the
information, especially with regard to drug usage, complies with
current legislation and standards of practice.

The
publisher's
policy is to use
**paper manufactured
from sustainable forests**

Produced by Longman Asia Ltd, Hong Kong
NPCC/01

INTRODUCTION

This anatomy book was produced in response to the publication in 1993 of *Tomorrow's Doctors*, by the General Medical Council. In its document the Council sought to promote a change in teaching philosophy by medical schools such that didactic teaching by staff was to be reduced, and self-directed learning by students encouraged. The pace and direction of study should be very much controlled by the individual student with staff involvement kept reasonably low-key. Students are therefore faced with the initially daunting task of sorting the large number of anatomical facts into what is crucially important to them to know and what is less important. There remains, however, a need for their teacher to ensure that the material under study is well presented and structured.

This book consists of a series of anatomical drawings arranged by region. Each drawing contains some basic or core anatomical information in the form of selected structures. The student should use these as a 'jumping off' point from which to explore the illustrated structures in more detail using, for example, an anatomical textbook, prosected specimen, model or computer software package. There are two principal functions to this book. Firstly, the active participation of the student in the learning process. Secondly, to promote the use of other learning media currently available in an anatomy teaching laboratory.

Each figure, with a few deliberate exceptions, has a number of leader lines on it with the corresponding labels arranged alphabetically at the foot of the page. The labels can be matched to the given leader lines and in addition the student may wish to identify other structures depending on their level of study. Some figures have more leader lines than labels as some structures can be labelled more than once e.g. a nerve may be indicated at both its proximal and distal ends. The student should be encouraged to colour the figures using the following convention: arteries — red, nerves — yellow, veins — blue and muscles — brown. In order to ensure the clarity of the figures it has been necessary to show some of the structures as solid black. The orientation of the figures has not been stated because it is in itself a learning exercise for students to recognise the orientation of certain structures out of situ.

The drawings have been chosen to provide the student with a wide selection of anatomical structures and we are extremely grateful to the very many undergraduates who aided us in this selection. We hope that new generations of students, whether they be medical, dental, paramedical or health science, will find this book a useful and enjoyable introduction to the learning of topographical anatomy.

I.L., F.K., J.S.
Edinburgh, 1996

CONTENTS

Section 1
HEAD AND NECK

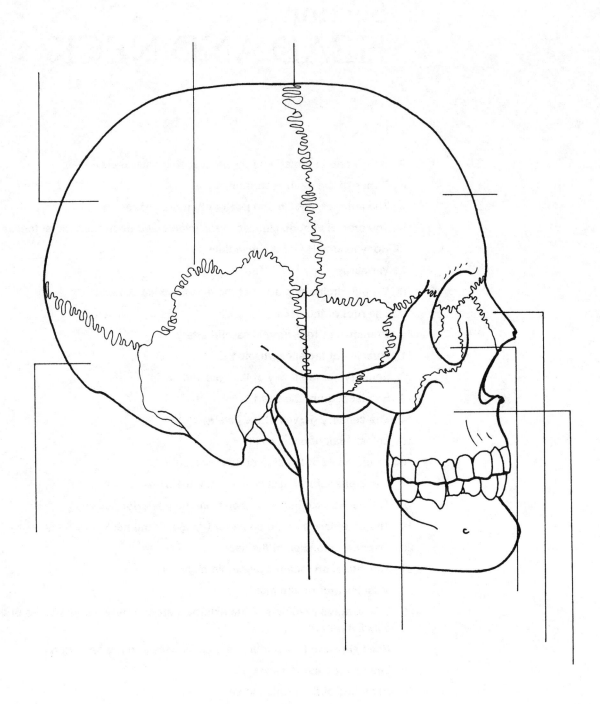

Coronal suture

Frontal bone

Lacrimal bone

Maxilla

Nasal bone

Occipital bone

Parietal bone

Pterion

Sphenoid bone

Squamosal suture

Zygomaticotemporal suture

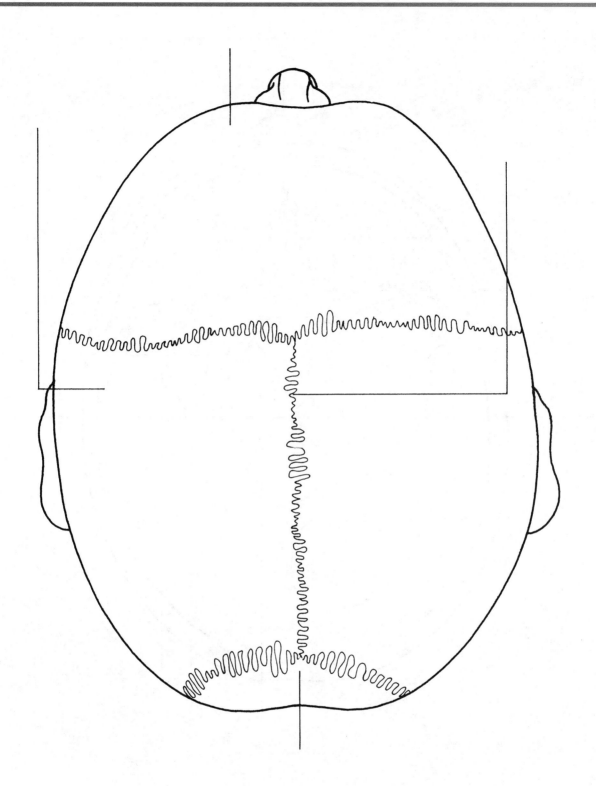

Frontal bone

Occipital bone

Parietal bone

Sagittal suture

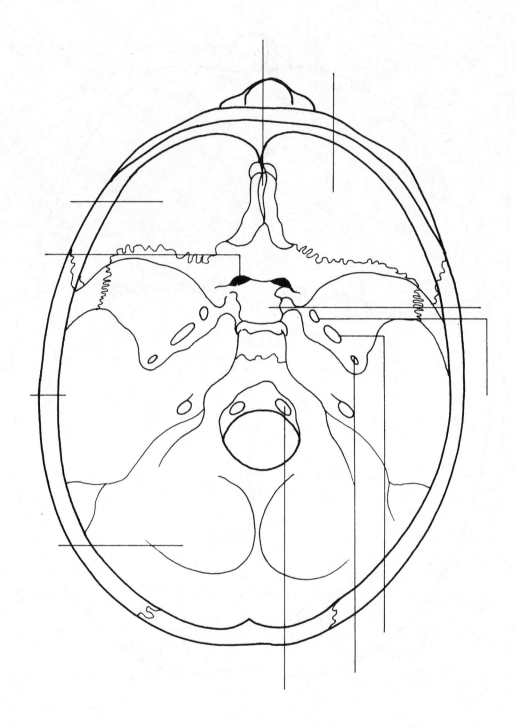

Anterior cranial fossa

Crista galli

Foramen ovale

Foramen rotundum

Foramen spinosum

Hypoglossal canal

Middle cranial fossa

Optic canal

Orbital plate of frontal bone

Pituitary fossa

Posterior cranial fossa

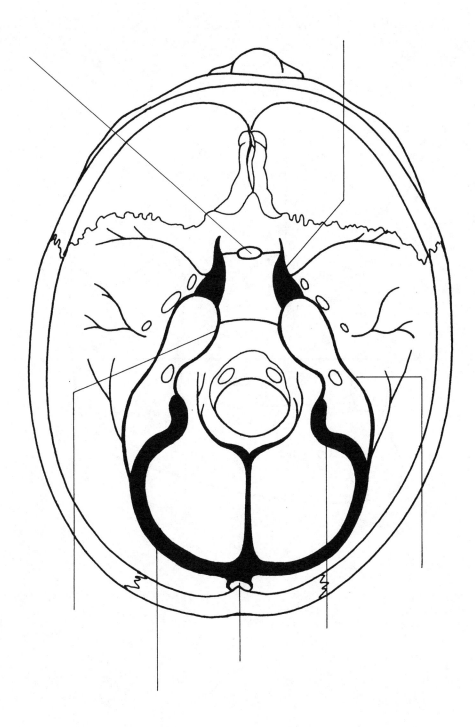

Cavernous sinus

Confluence of sinuses

Inferior petrosal sinus

Pituitary fossa

Sigmoid sinus

Superior petrosal sinus

Transverse sinus

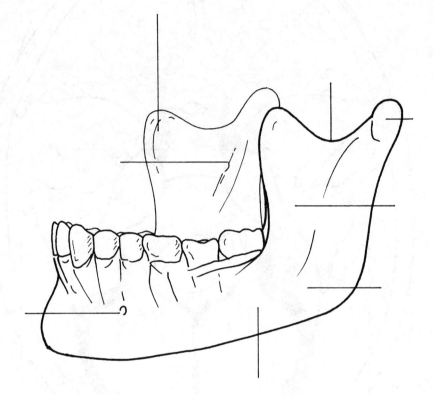

Angle of mandible

Body of mandible

Condyle (head of mandible)

Coronoid process

Mandibular foramen

Mandibular notch

Mental foramen

Ramus

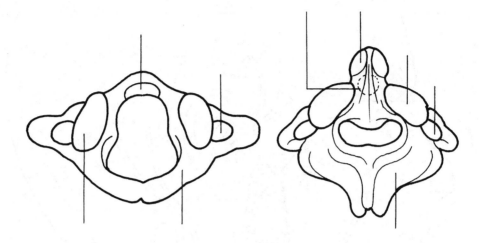

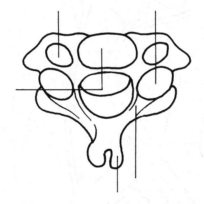

Bifurcation of spine

Concave superior articular facet

Facet for articulation with
odontoid process of axis

Facet for transverse ligament

Flat superior articular facet

Foramen transversarium

Lamina

Odontoid process

Vertebral body

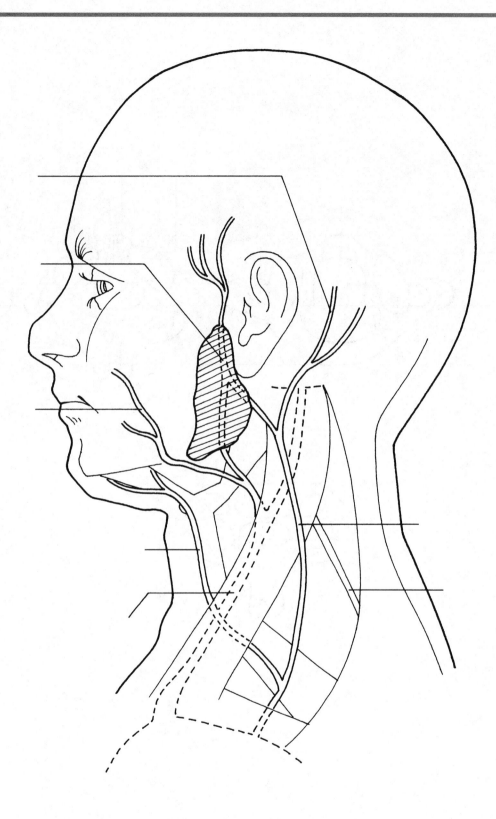

Anterior jugular vein   Posterior auricular vein

External jugular vein   Retromandibular vein

Facial vein   Spinal accessory nerve

Internal jugular vein

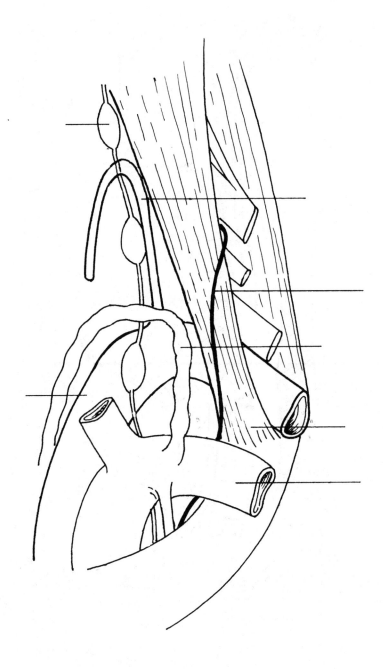

Inferior thyroid artery

Middle cervical sympathetic ganglion

Phrenic nerve

Scalenus anterior

Subclavian vein

Subclavian artery

Thoracic duct

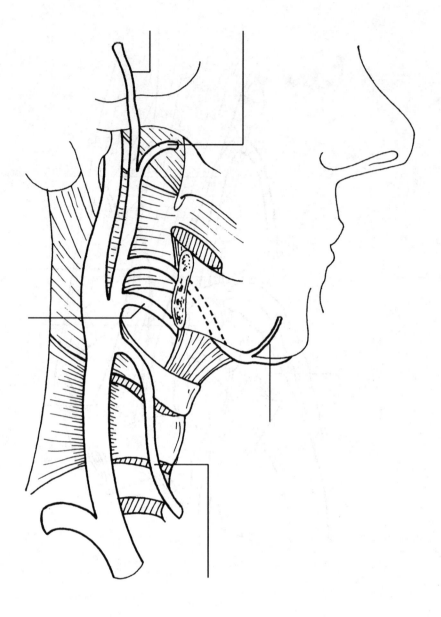

Facial artery

Lingual artery

Maxillary artery

Superficial temporal artery

Superior thyroid artery

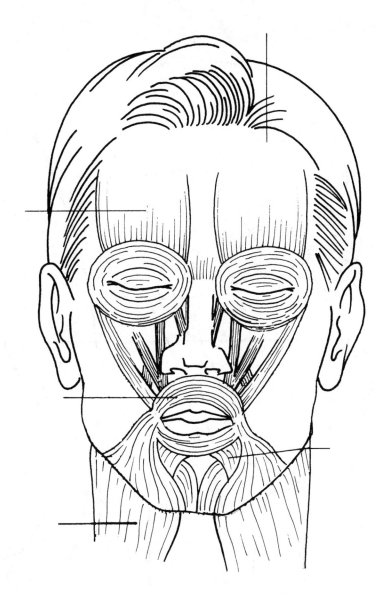

Depressor labii inferioris

Epicranial aponeurosis

Frontalis

Orbicularis oris

Platysma

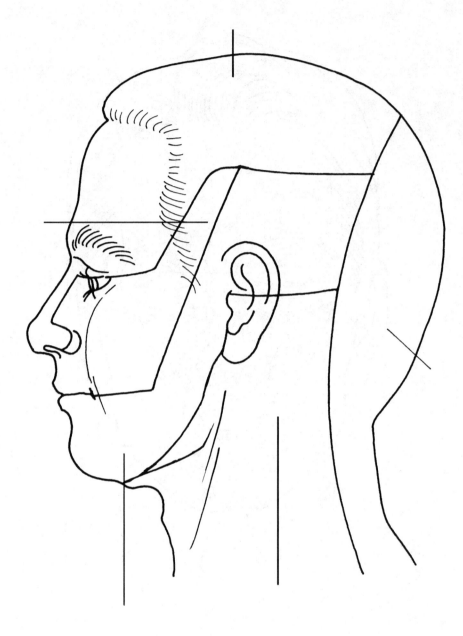

Dorsal rami of cervical nerve

Mandibular division of trigeminal nerve

Maxillary division of trigeminal nerve

Ophthalmic division of trigeminal nerve

Ventral rami of cervical nerve

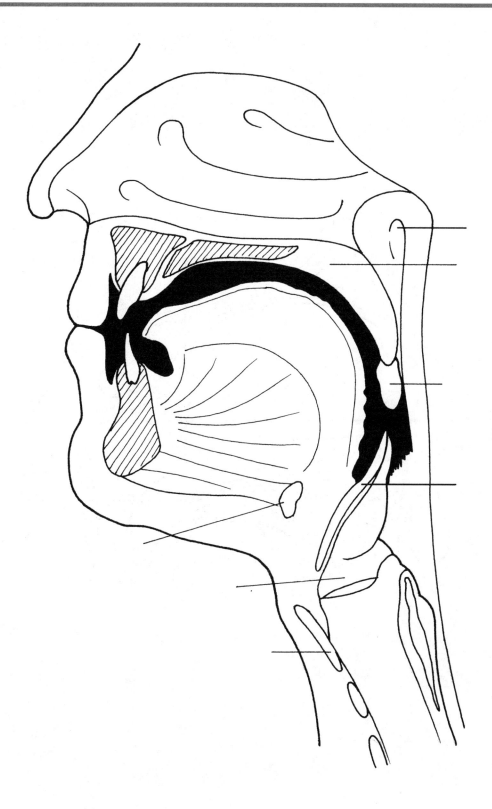

Auditory tube

Body of hyoid bone

Epiglottis

Palatine tonsil

Soft palate

Thyroid cartilage

Vestibule of larynx

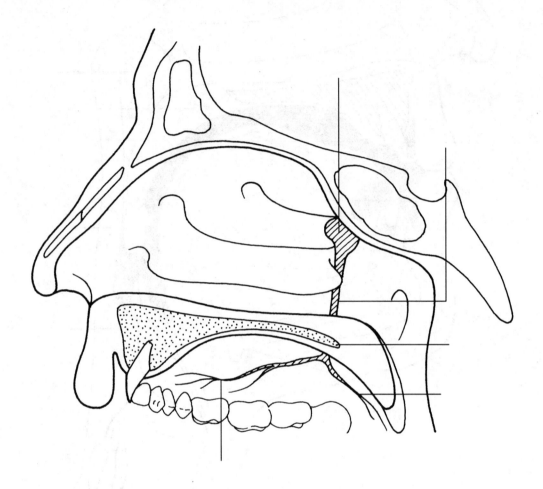

Greater palatine nerve

Lesser palatine nerve

Nerve in palatine canal

Palatine bone

Sphenopalatine foramen

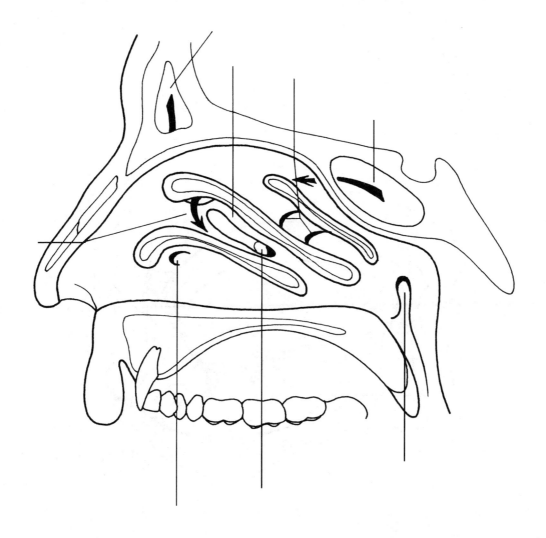

Auditory tube

Bulla ethmoidalis

Frontal sinus

Nasolacrimal duct

Opening of frontal air sinus &
anterior ethmoidal air sinus

Opening of maxillary air sinus

Opening of posterior ethmoidal
air sinus

Opening of sphenoidal air sinus

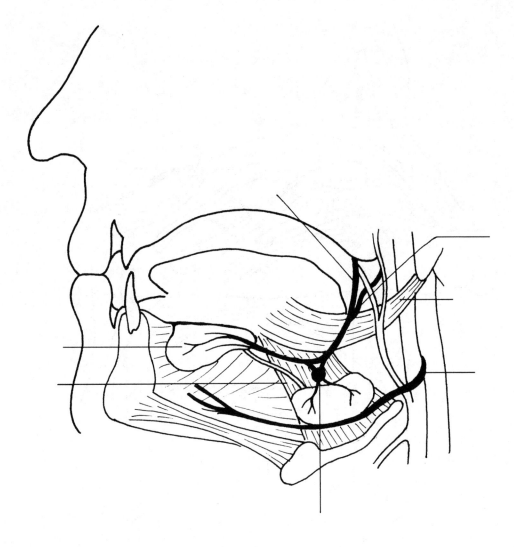

Chorda tympani

Hyoglossus muscle

Hypoglossal nerve

Lingual nerve

Styloglossus muscle

Sublingual gland

Submandibular ganglion

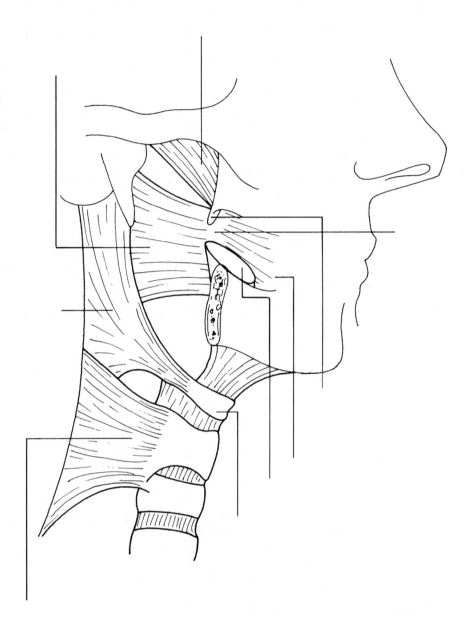

Buccinator muscle

Hyoid bone

Inferior constrictor

Medial pterygoid

Middle constrictor

Pterygoid hamulus

Pterygomandibular raphe

Superior constrictor

Tensor veli palatini

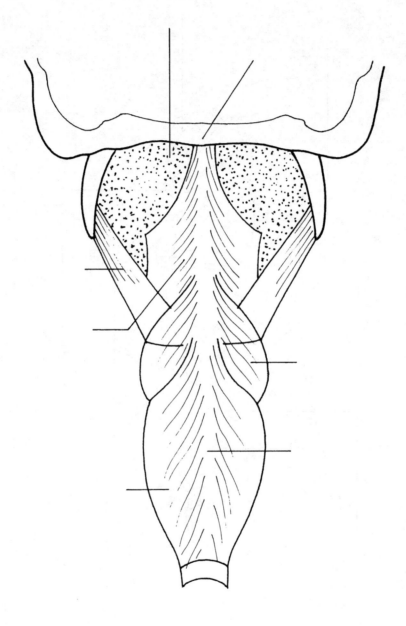

Inferior constrictor

Middle constrictor

Midline raphe

Pharyngeal tubercle

Pharyngobasilar fascia

Stylopharyngeus

Superior constrictor

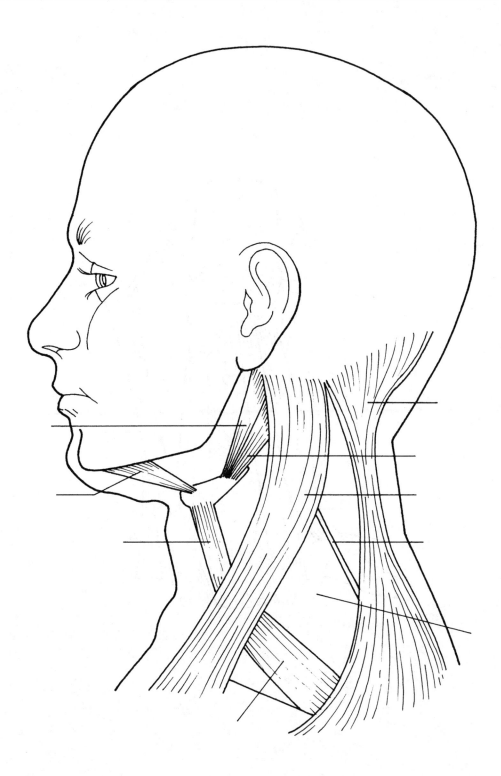

Anterior digastric muscle

Inferior belly of omohyoid muscle

Posterior digastric muscle

Prevertebral fascia

Spinal accessory nerve

Sternocleidomastoid muscle

Stylohyoid muscle

Superior belly of omohyoid muscle

Trapezius

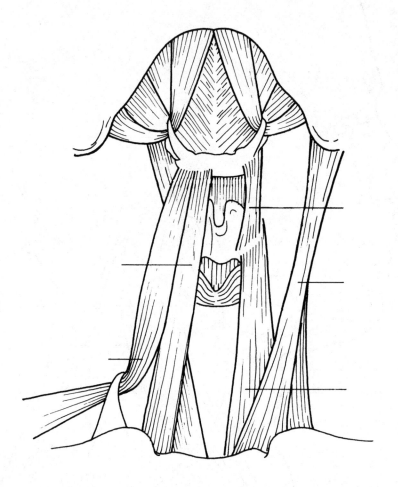

Sternocleidomastoid muscle

Sternohyoid muscle

Sternothyroid muscle

Superior belly of omohyoid muscle

Thyrohyoid muscle

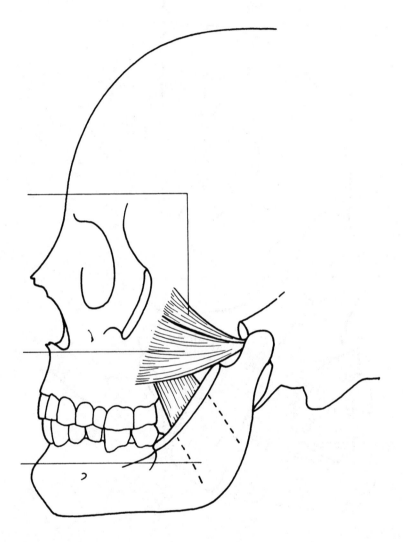

Lateral pterygoid muscle
(lower head)

Lateral pterygoid muscle
(upper head)

Medial pterygoid muscle

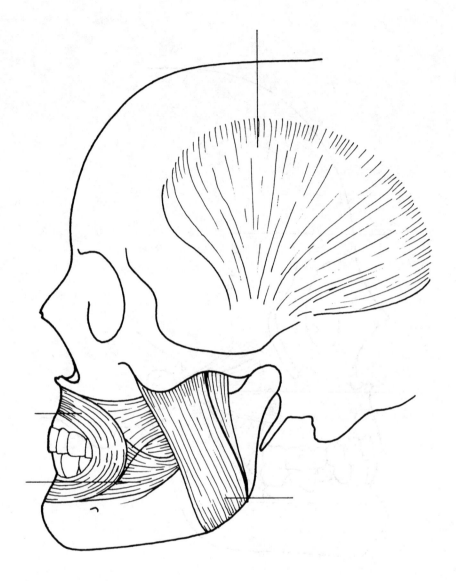

Buccinator

Masseter

Orbicularis oris

Temporalis muscle

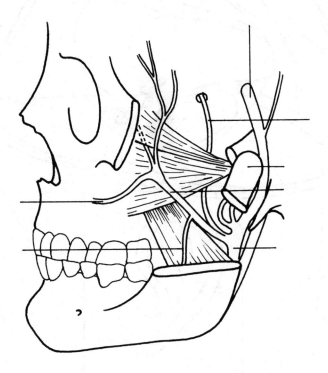

Condyle of mandible

External carotid artery

Inferior alveolar artery

Maxillary artery

Middle meningeal artery

Superficial temporal artery

Superior alveolar artery

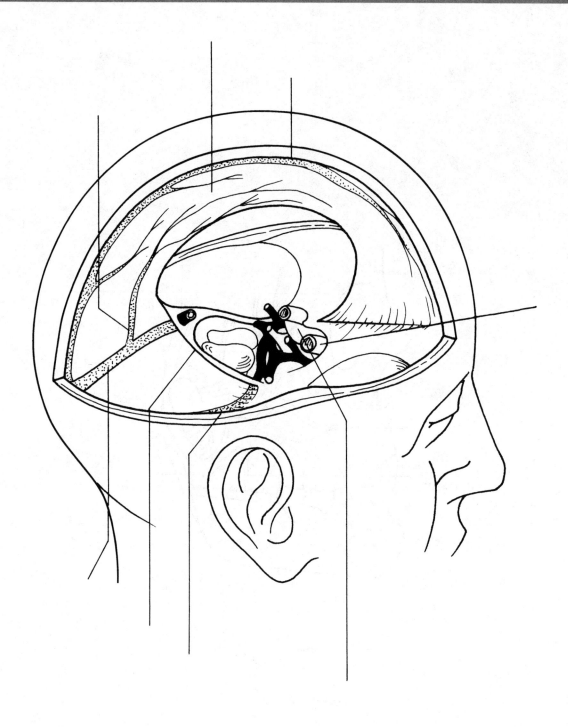

Falx cerebri

Free margin of tentorium

Inferior sagittal sinus

Optic nerve

Pituitary fossa

Straight sinus

Superior sagittal sinus

Transverse sinus

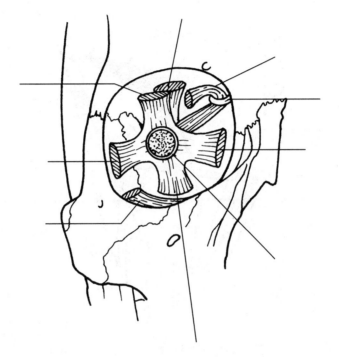

Fibrous ring

Inferior oblique

Inferior rectus

Levator palpabrae superioris

Medial rectus

Superior oblique

Superior rectus

Trochlea

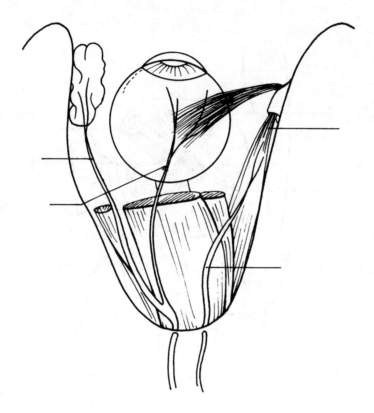

Frontal nerve

Lacrimal nerve

Superior oblique muscle

Trochlear nerve

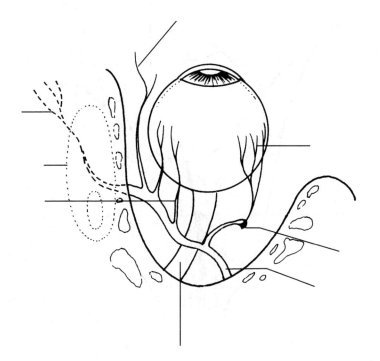

Ciliary ganglion

Ethmoidal air sinuses

External nasal nerve

Infratrochlear nerve

Long ciliary nerves

Nasociliary nerve

Optic nerve

Short ciliary nerves

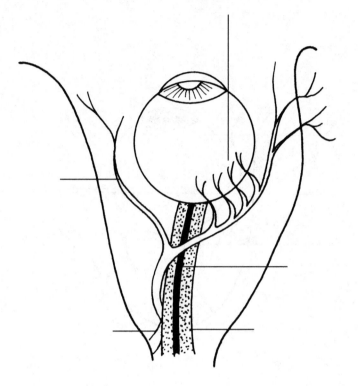

Central artery

Ciliary arteries

Lacrimal artery

Ophthalmic artery

Optic nerve

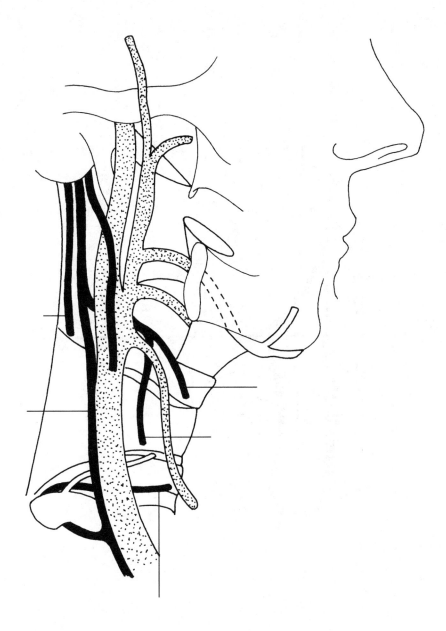

Accessory nerve

External laryngeal nerve

Internal laryngeal nerve

Right recurrent laryngeal nerve

Vagus nerve

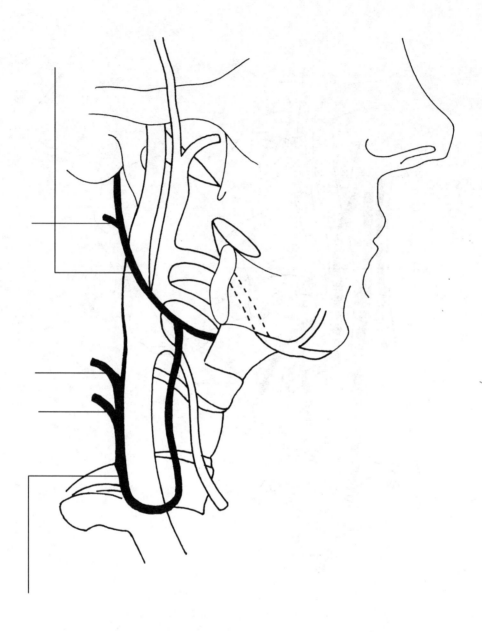

Ansa cervicalis

Hypoglossal nerve

Ventral ramus C1

Ventral ramus C2

Ventral ramus C3

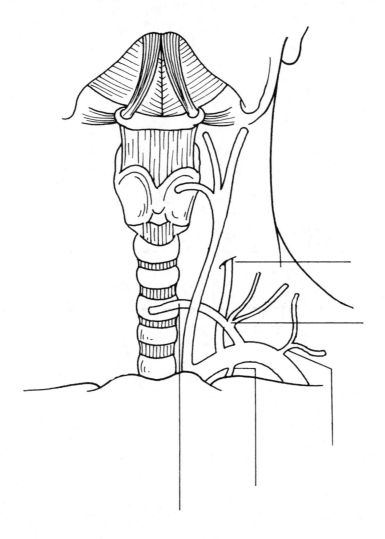

Costocervical trunk

Inferior thyroid artery

Internal thoracic artery

Thyrocervical trunk

Vertebral artery

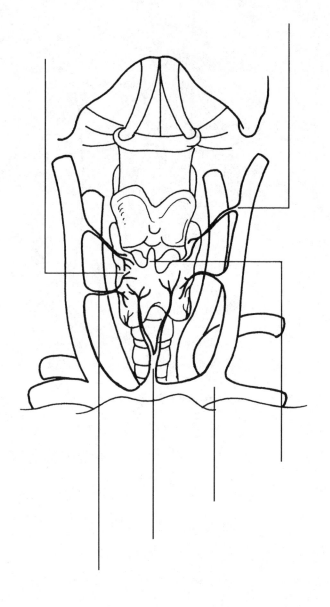

Inferior thyroid veins

Lateral lobe of thyroid

Left brachiocephalic vein

Middle thyroid vein

Pyramidal lobe

Superior thyroid vein

Section 2
THORAX

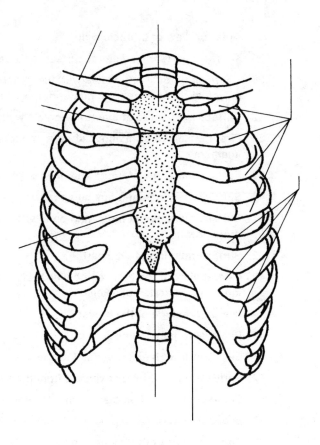

2nd rib   Manubriosternal joint

12th rib (floating)   Manubrium

Body of sternum   Ribs

Clavicle   Xiphoid process

Costal cartilages

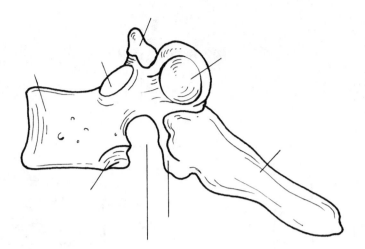

A

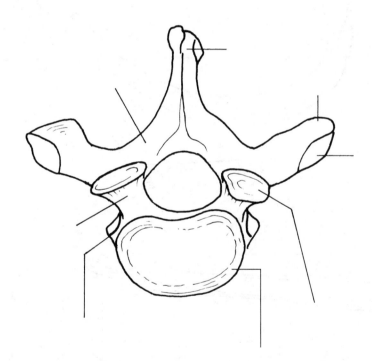

B

Body of vertebra	Spinous process
Facet for tubercle of rib	Superior articular facet
Inferior articular facet	Transverse process
Inferior vertebral notch	Upper and lower articular facets for heads of ribs
Lamina	
Pedicle	

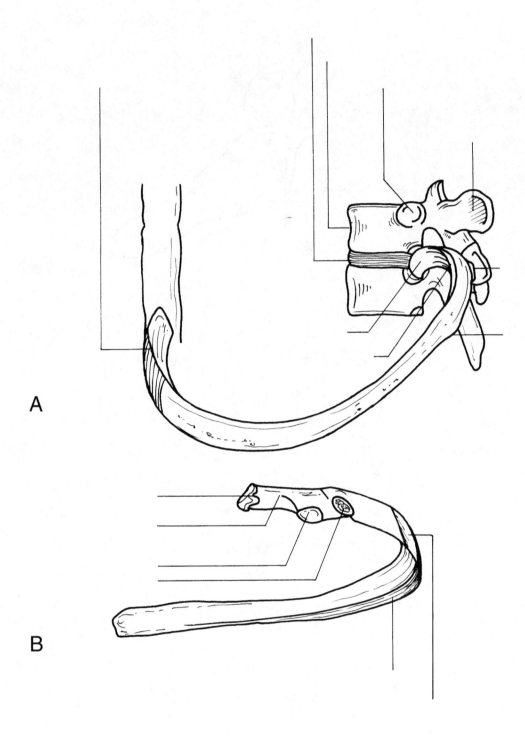

A

B

Annulus fibrosus

Attachment of lateral
costotransverse ligament

Costal cartilage

Costal groove

Demifacets for heads of ribs

Facet for tubercle of ribs

Head of rib with two articular
demifacets

Neck of rib

Rib angle

Tubercle of rib

Vertebral body

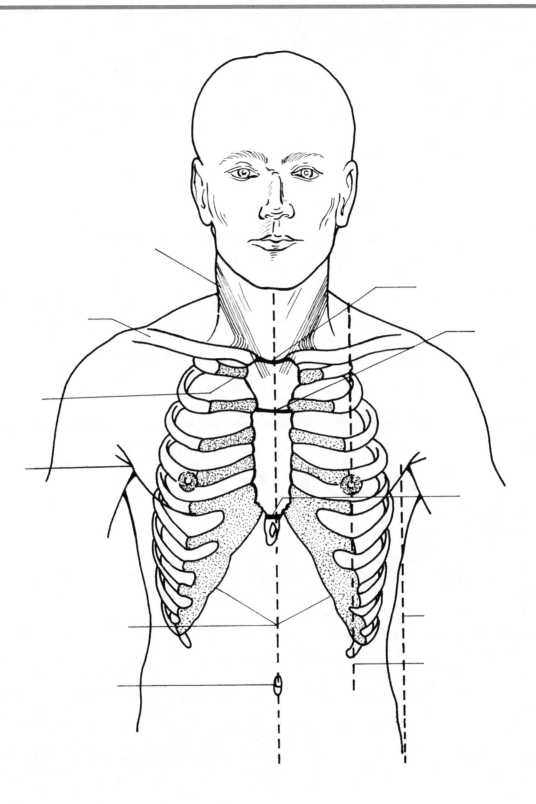

1st costal cartilage

Anterior axillary fold

Anterior axillary line

Costal margin

Lateral end of clavicle

Midclavicular line

Sternal angle

Sternocleidomastoid muscle

Suprasternal notch

Umbilicus on midline

Xiphisternal joint

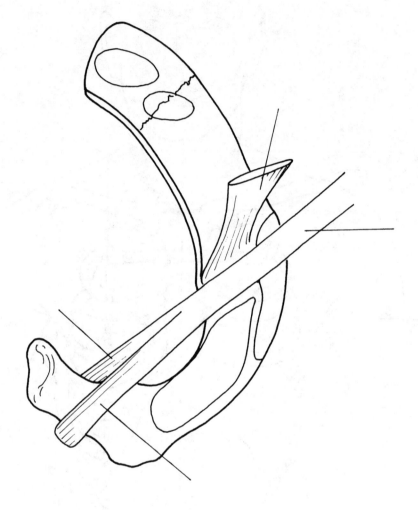

Anterior (ventral) ramus C8

Anterior (ventral) ramus T1

Lower trunk of brachial plexus

Scalenus anterior

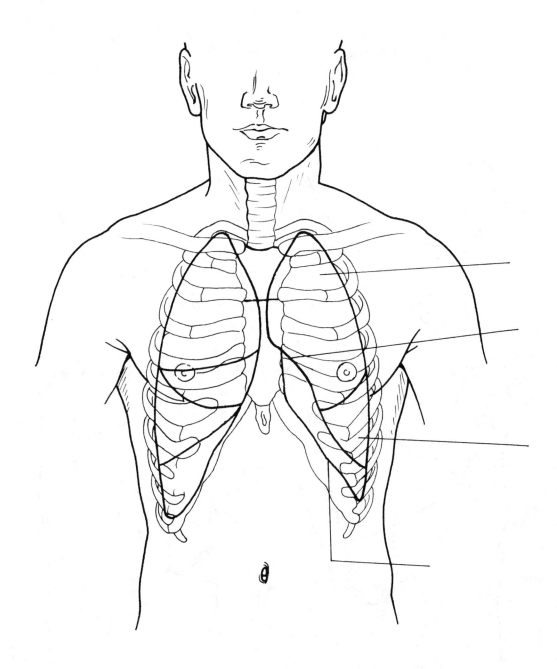

Cardiac notch

Line of pleural reflection

Lower (inferior) lobe

Upper (superior) lobe

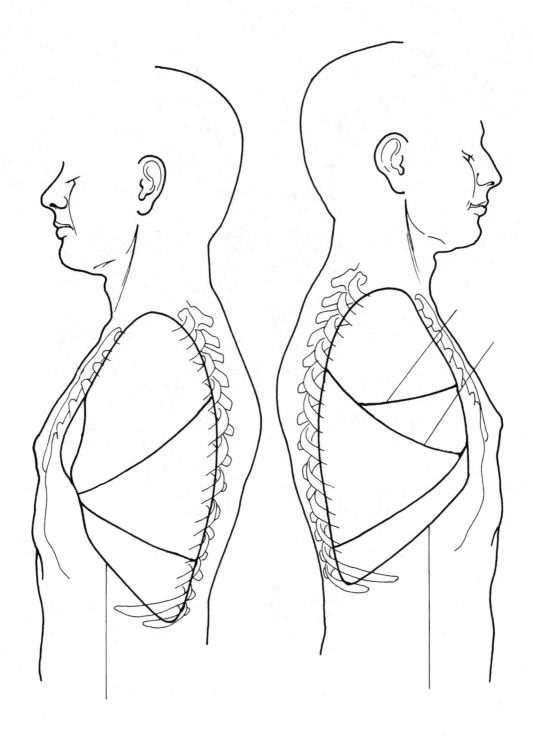

Horizontal fissure

Lower border of pleura

Oblique fissure

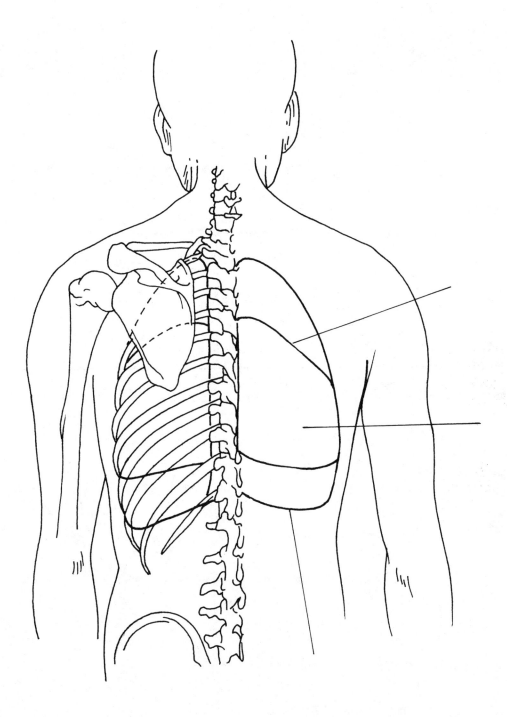

Lower border of pleura

Lower (inferior) lobe

Oblique fissure

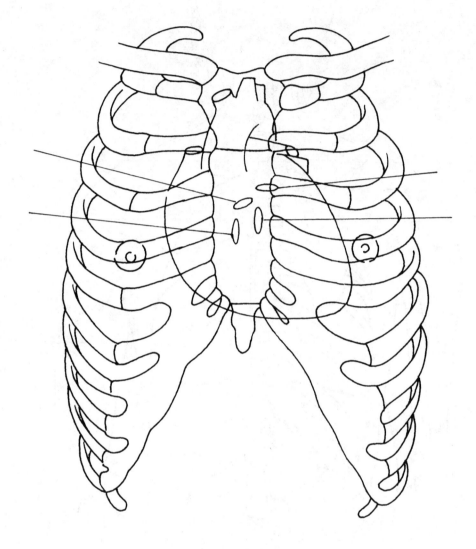

Aortic valve

Mitral valve

Pulmonary valve

Tricuspid valve

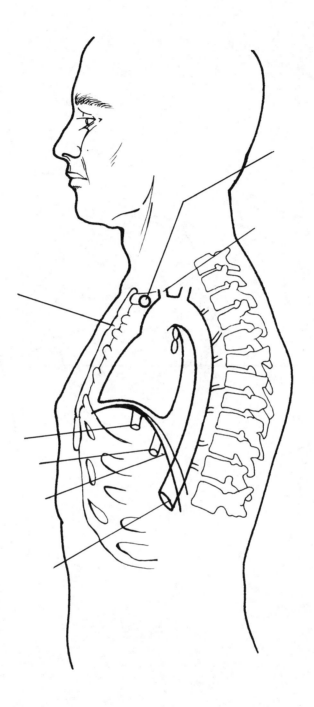

Aorta

Diaphragm

Inferior vena cava

Left brachiocephalic vein

Left common carotid artery

Oesophagus

Sternal angle

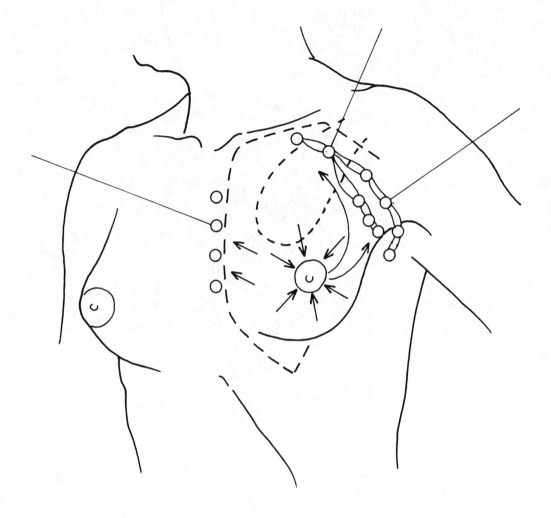

Apical axillary lymph node

Parasternal lymph node

Pectoral axillary lymph node

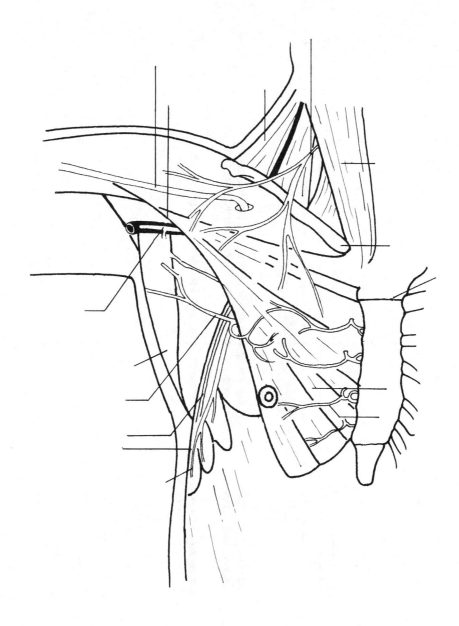

Anterior cutaneous branch of intercostal nerve

Axillary artery

Cephalic vein

Digitation of serratus anterior

Intercostobrachial nerve

Latissimus dorsi

Long thoracic nerve

Manibriosternal joint

Medial cutaneous nerve of forearm

Medial end of clavicle

Pectoralis major

Sternocleidomastoid

Supraclavicular nerves

Thoracodorsal nerve

Trapezius

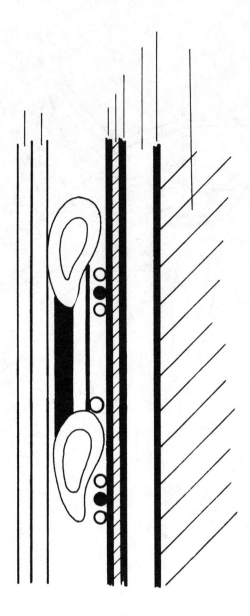

Endothoracic fascia	Parietal pleura
Fascia	Pleural cavity
Innermost layer of intercostal muscle	Skin
Lung	Visceral pleura

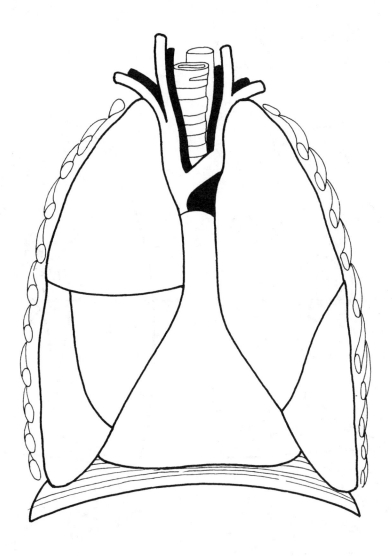

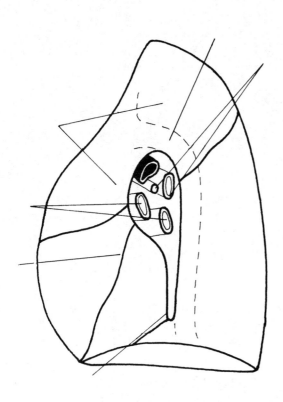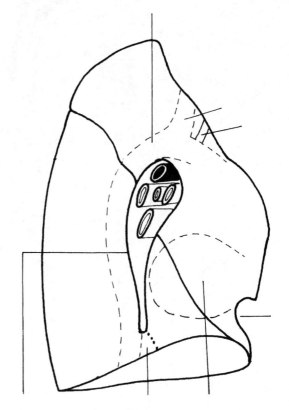

Arch of aorta

Azygos vein

Bronchus

Cardiac notch

Depression for left ventricle

Groove for left subclavian artery

Left common carotid artery

Oblique fissure

Oesophagus

Pulmonary ligament

Pulmonary veins

Upper (superior) lobe

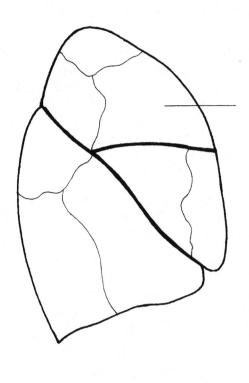
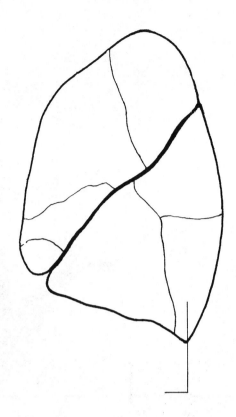
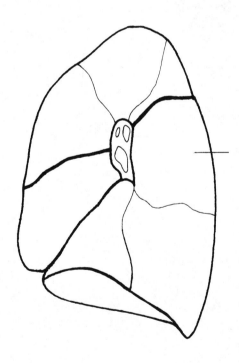
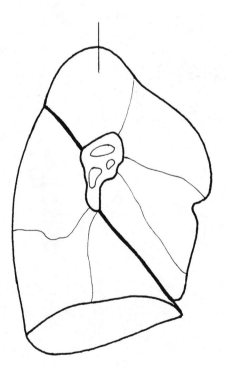

Anterior

Apical posterior

Lateral basal

Superior (apical) of inferior lobe

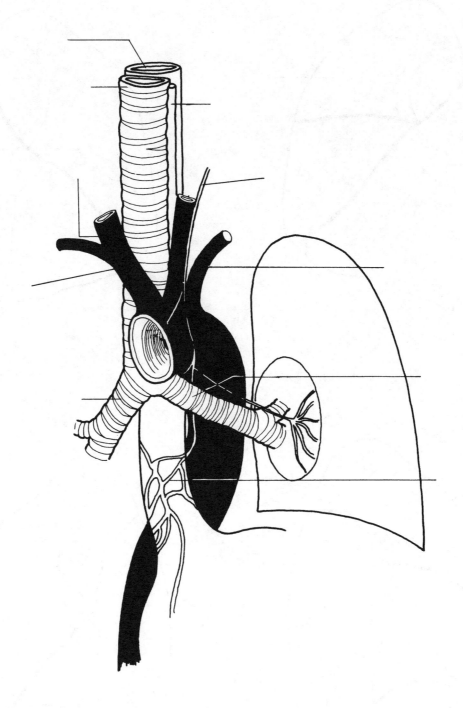

Brachiocephalic artery

Left principal bronchus

Left subclavian artery

Left vagus nerve

Oesophageal plexus

Oesophagus

Right common carotid artery

Right principal bronchus

Thoracic duct

Trachea

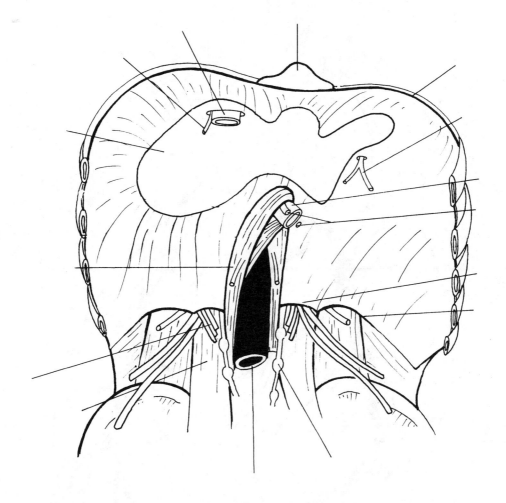

Abdominal aorta

Anterior and posterior vagal trunks

Central tendon

Inferior vena cava

Lateral arcuate ligament

Left dome of the diaphragm

Left phrenic nerve

Medial arcuate ligament

Oesophagus

Psoas major

Right phrenic nerve

Splanchnic nerves

Sympathetic trunk

Xiphoid process

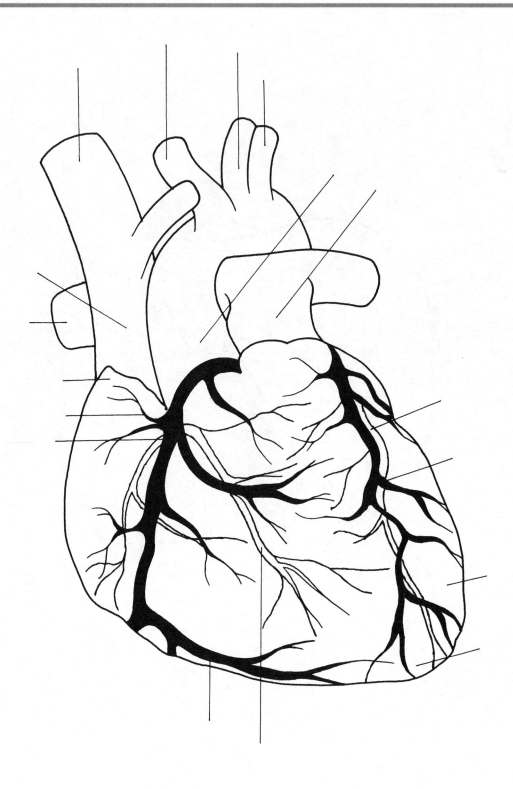

Anterior cardiac vein

Anterior interventricular artery

Apex

Ascending aorta

Brachiocephalic artery

Branch to the sinuatrial node

Great cardiac vein

Left common carotid artery

Left subclavian artery

Left ventricle

Marginal artery

Pulmonary trunk

Right auricle

Right brachiocephalic vein

Right coronary artery

Right pulmonary artery

Superior vena cava

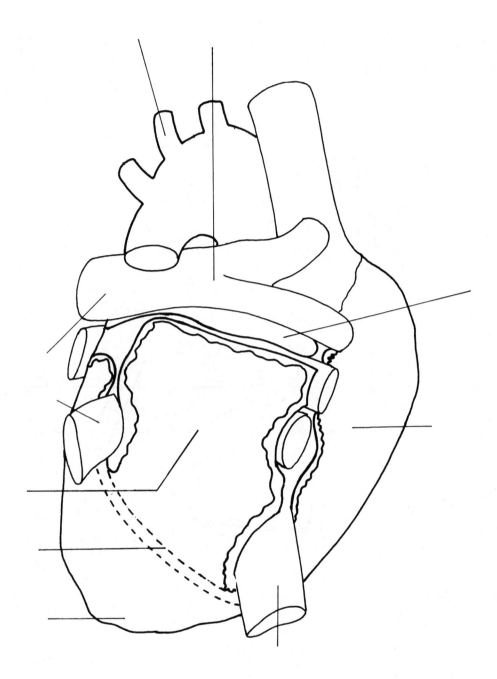

Coronary sinus

Inferior vena cava

Left common carotid artery

Left pulmonary artery

Left pulmonary vein

Left ventricle

Oblique sinus of pericardium

Right atrium

Right pulmonary artery

Transverse sinus of pericardium

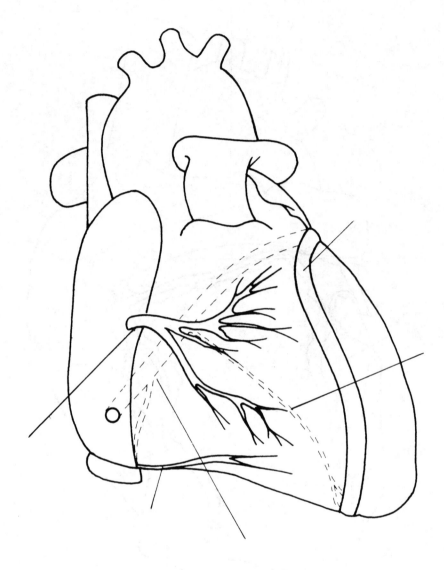

Anterior cardiac vein

Coronary sinus

Great cardiac vein

Middle cardiac vein

Small cardiac vein

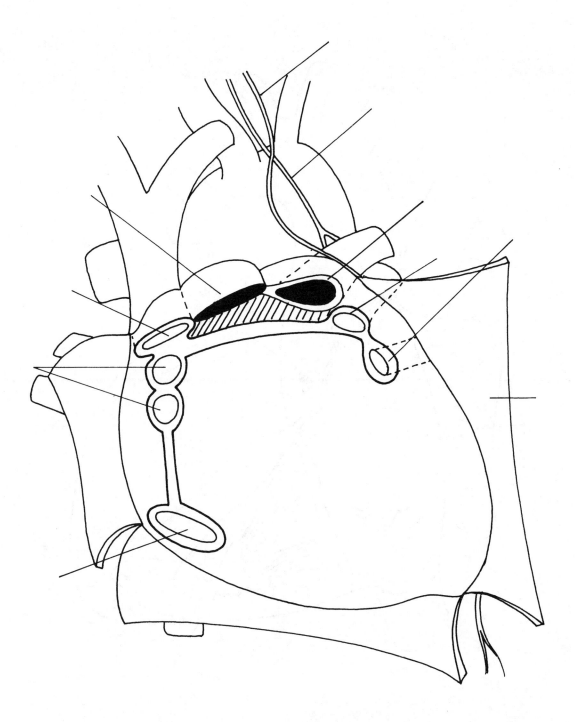

Ascending aorta

Inferior vena cava

Left and right pulmonary veins

Left phrenic nerve

Left vagus nerve

Parietal layer of serous pericardium

Pulmonary trunk

Superior vena cava

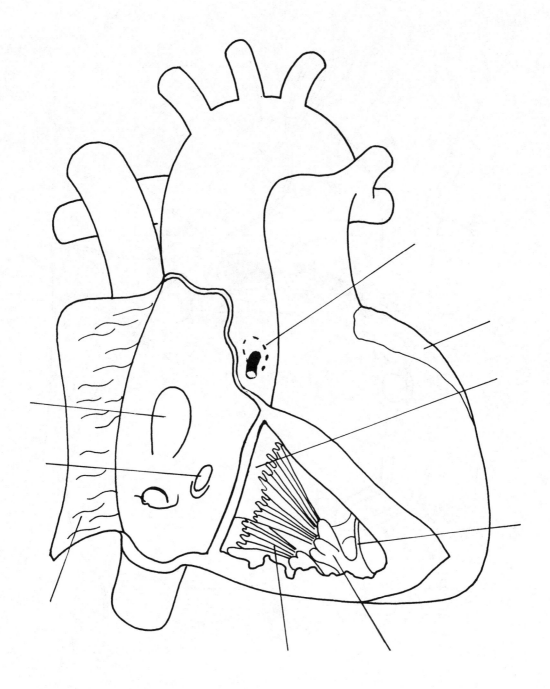

Anterior aortic sinus and origin of right coronary artery

Anterior cusp of tricuspid valve

Chordae tendineae

Coronary sinus

Fossa ovalis

Left auricle

Musculi pectinati

Papillary muscle

Trabecula septomarginalis

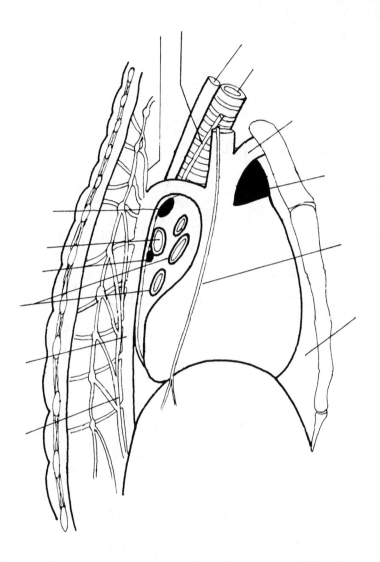

Anterior mediastinum

Ascending aorta

Azygos vein

Bronchial artery

Greater splanchnic nerve

Left brachiocephalic vein

Oesophagus

Pulmonary arteries

Pulmonary veins

Right bronchus

Right phrenic nerve

Right superior intercostal vein

Right vagus nerve

Trachea

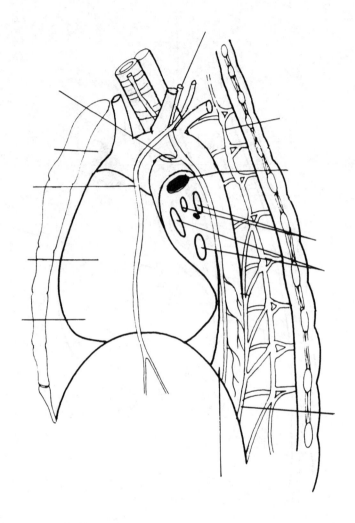

Anterior mediastinum

Greater splanchnic nerve

Left bronchus

Left phrenic nerve

Left pulmonary artery

Left pulmonary veins

Left recurrent laryngeal nerve

Left vagus nerve

Left ventricle covered by
pericardium

Oesophagus

Pericardium

Sympathetic trunk

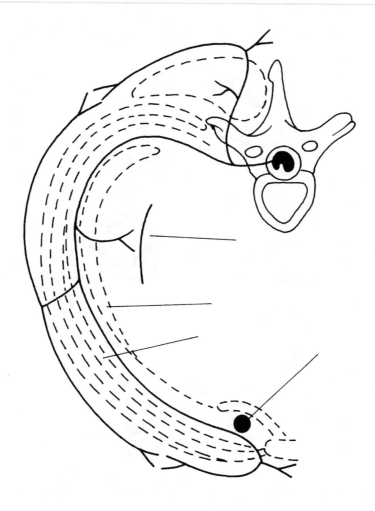

Innermost intercostal muscle

Internal intercostal muscle

Internal thoracic artery

Parietal pleura

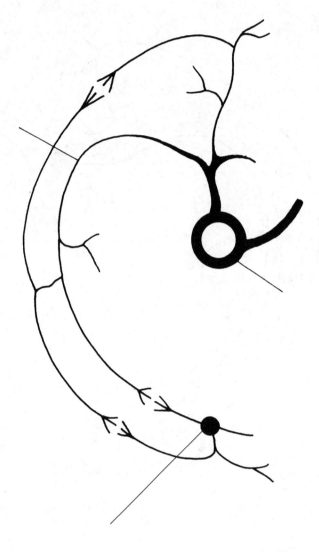

Internal thoracic artery

Posterior intercostal artery

Thoracic aorta

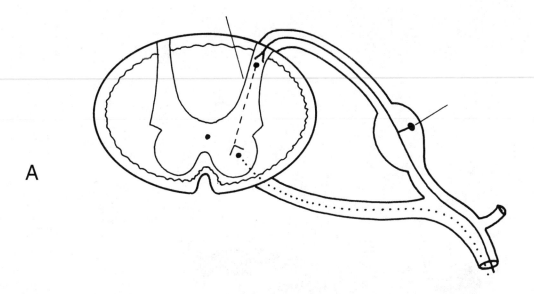

A

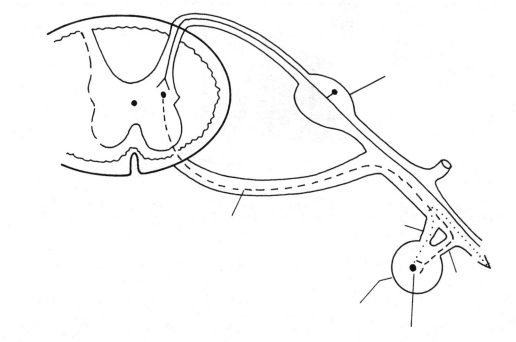

B

Efferent sympathetic fibres in
ventral root

Gray ramus communicans

Posterior (dorsal) horn of grey
matter

Posterior (dorsal) root ganglion

Pseudounipolar (sensory)
neurone

Sympathetic ganglion

Synapse in sympathetic ganglion

White ramus communicans

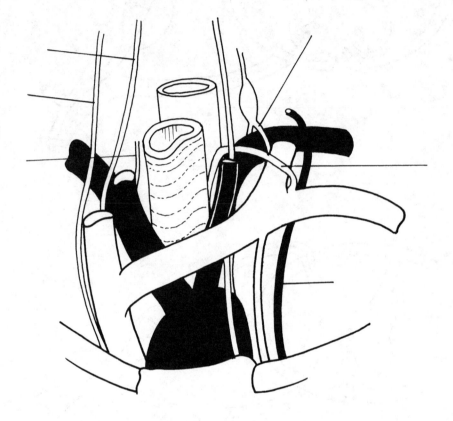

Ansa subclavia

Internal thoracic artery

Right phrenic nerve

Right recurrent laryngeal nerve

Right vagus nerve

Thoracic duct

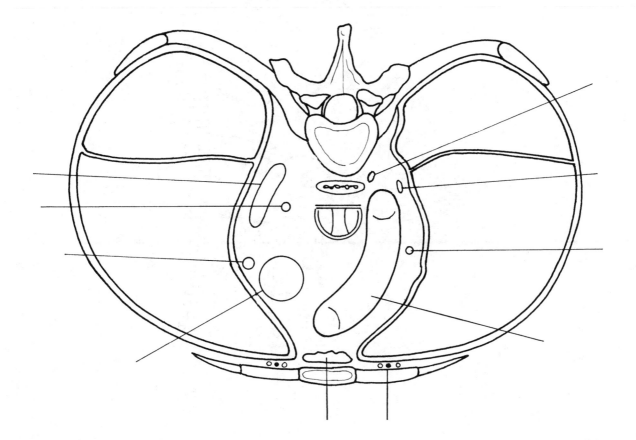

Arch of aorta (cut)	Right phrenic nerve
Azygos vein	Right vagus nerve
Left internal thoracic artery	Thoracic duct
Left phrenic nerve	Thymus
Left vagus nerve	Superior vena cava

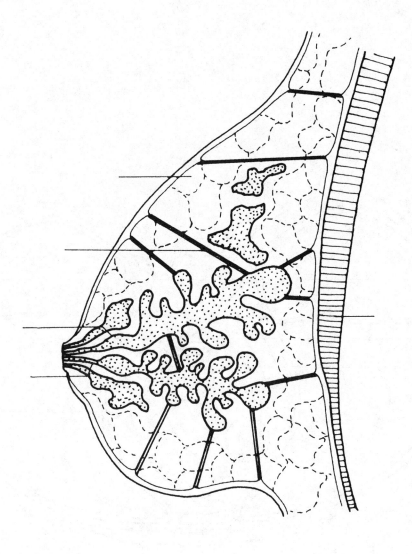

Fat

Lactiferous duct

Lactiferous sinus

Pectoralis major muscle

Suspensory ligament

Section 3
UPPER LIMB

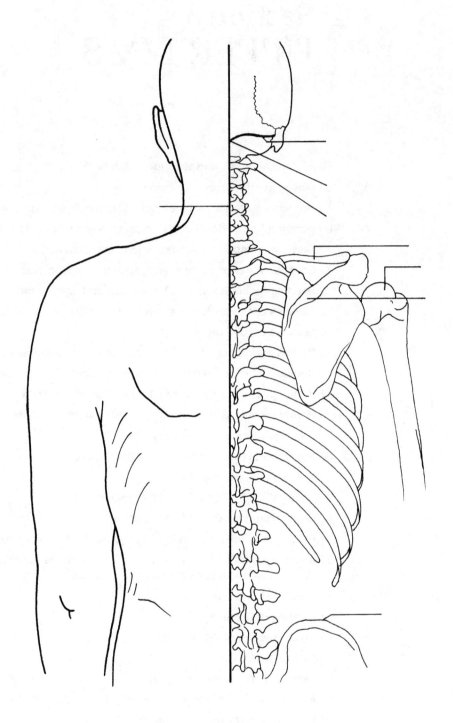

Atlas

Cervical vertebra

Clavicle

External occipital protruberance

Head of humerus

Iliac crest

Spine of scapula

Superior nuchal line

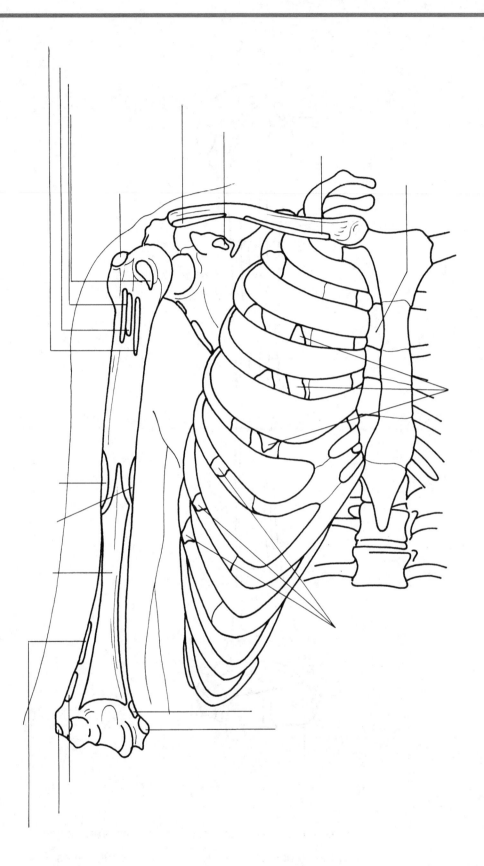

Brachialis	Deltoid	Pronator teres
Brachioradialis	Extensor carpi radialis longus	Serratus anterior
Common extensor tendon	Latissimus dorsi	Subscapularis
Common flexor tendon	Pectoralis major	Supraspinatus
Coracobrachialis	Pectoralis minor	Teres major

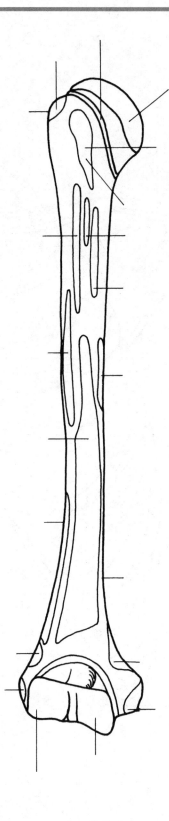

Brachialis

Capitulum

Capsule of shoulder joint

Common extensor tendon

Common flexor tendon

Coracobrachialis

Deltoid tuberosity

Extensor carpi radialis longus

Greater tuberosity

Head of humerus

Lateral supracondylar ridge

Latissimus dorsi

Lesser tuberosity

Medial supracondylar ridge

Pectoralis major

Pronator teres

Subscapularis

Supraspinatus

Teres major

Trochlea

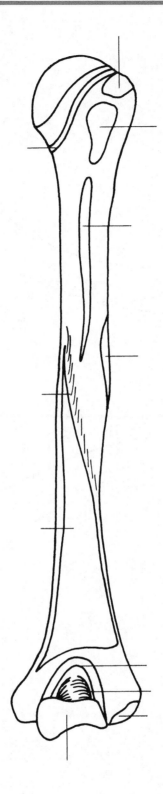

Anconeus

Capsule of elbow joint

Capsule of shoulder joint

Deltoid

Infraspinatus

Lateral head of triceps

Medial head of triceps

Olecranon fossa

Teres minor

Trochlea

Spiral groove

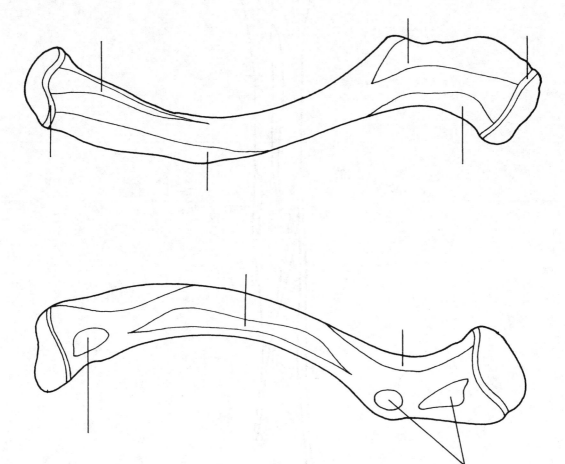

Capsule of acromioclavicular joint   Pectoralis major

Capsule of sternoclavicular joint   Sternocleidomastoid

Coracoclavicular ligament   Subclavius

Costoclavicular ligament   Trapezius

Deltoid

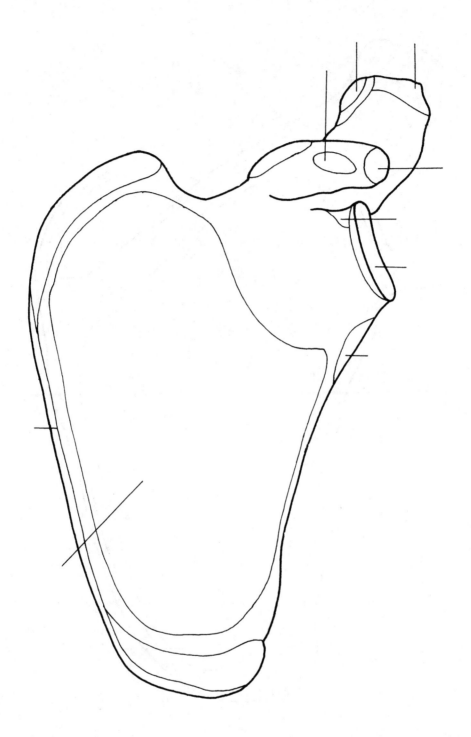

Articular surface for clavicle

Deltoid

Glenoid fossa

Long head of triceps

Pectoralis minor

Serratus anterior

Short head of biceps

Subscapularis or subscapular fossa

Supraglenoid tubercle

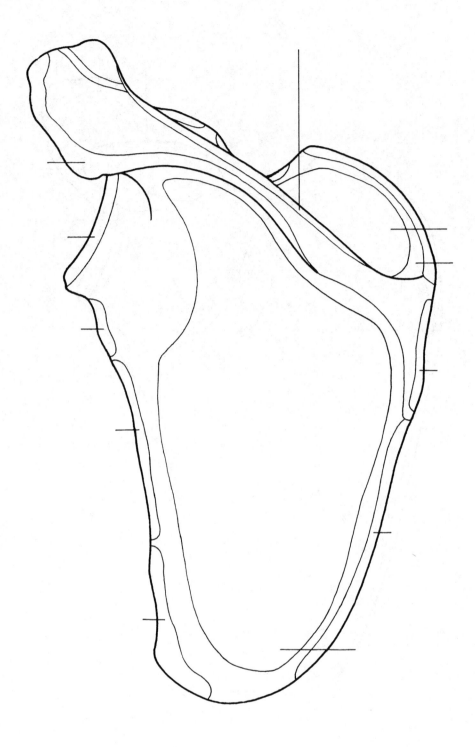

Deltoid

Glenoid fossa

Infraspinatus

Levator scapulae

Rhomboid major

Rhomboid minor

Supraspinatus

Teres major

Teres minor

Trapezius

Triceps (long head)

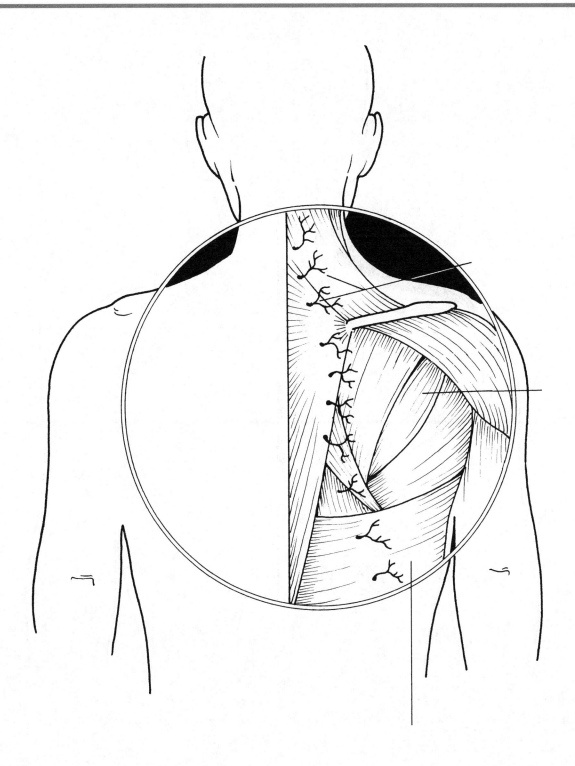

Dorsal (posterior) rami of spinal
nerves

Latissimus dorsi

Teres minor

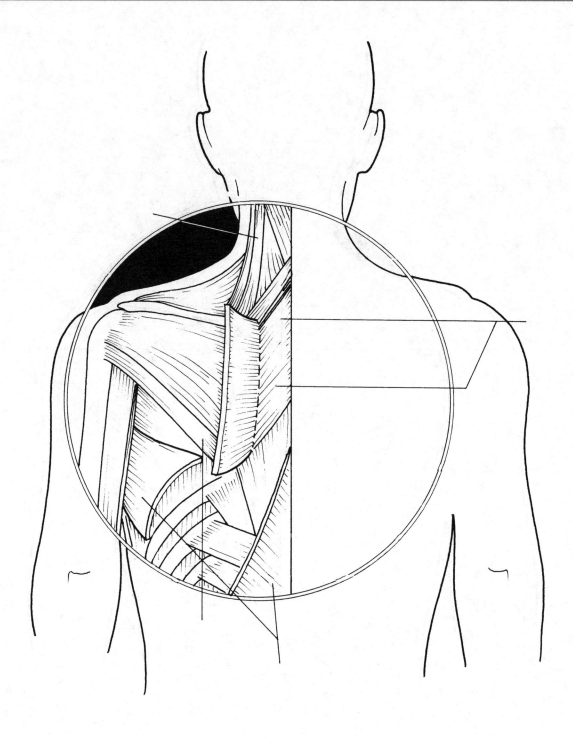

Latissimus dorsi

Levator scapulae

Rhomboid major

Teres minor

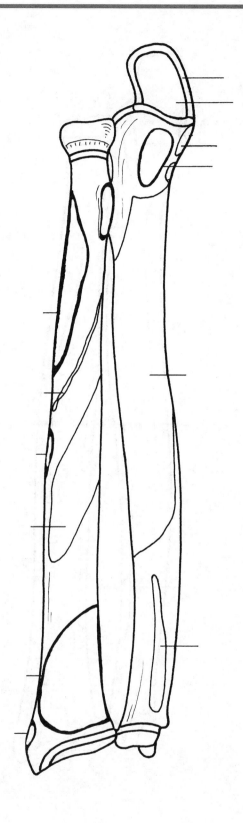

Brachialis

Brachioradialis

Capsule of elbow joint

Flexor digitorum profundus

Flexor digitorum superficialis

Flexor pollicis longus

Olecranon process

Pronator teres

Pronator quadratus

Supinator

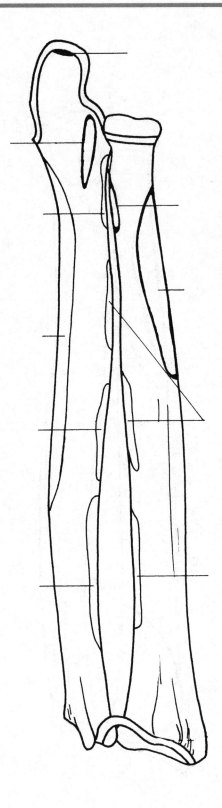

Abductor pollicis longus

Anconeus

Biceps

Extensor indicis

Extensor pollicis brevis

Extensor pollicis longus

Flexor digitorum profundus

Supinator

Triceps

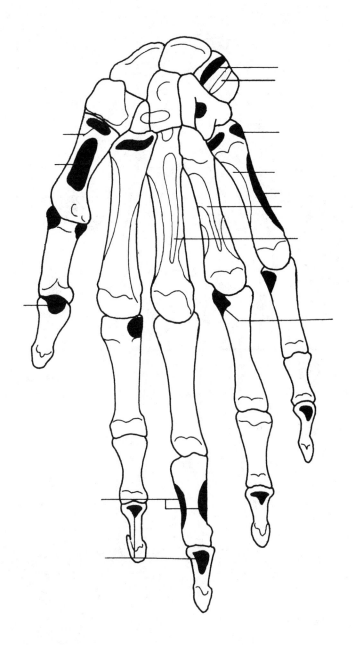

Abductor digiti minimi

Abductor pollicis longus

Adductor pollicis (transverse head)

Flexor carpi ulnaris

Flexor digitorum profundus

Flexor digitorum superficialis

Flexor pollicis longus

Opponens pollicis

Palmar interossei

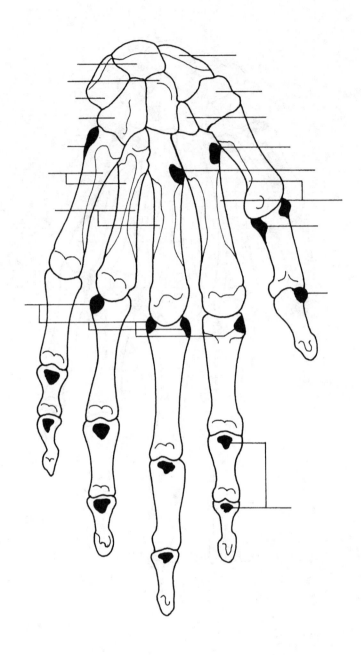

Adductor pollicis

Capitate

Dorsal interossei

Extensor carpi radialis brevis

Extensor carpi radialis longus

Extensor carpi ulnaris

Extensor digitorum

Extensor pollicis longus

Hamate

Lunate

Scaphoid

Trapezium

Trapezoid

Triquetral

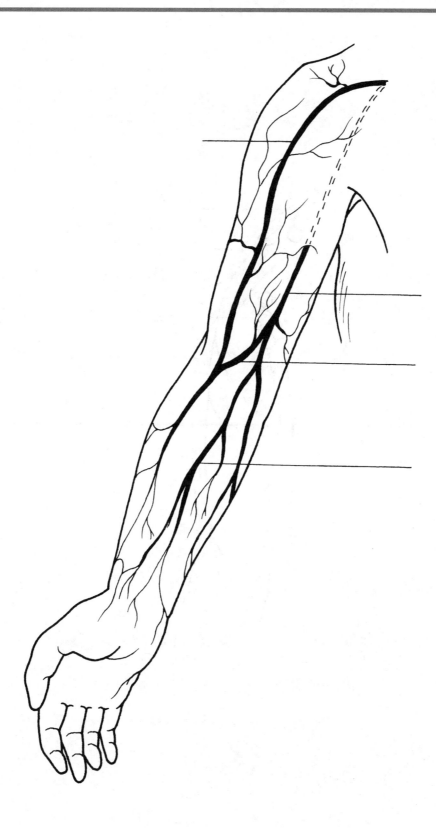

Anterior median vein of forearm

Basilic vein

Cephalic vein

Median cubital vein

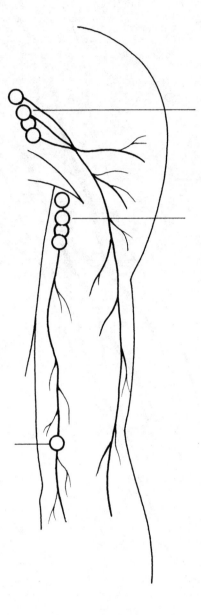

Axillary nodes

Infraclavicular nodes

Supratrochlear node

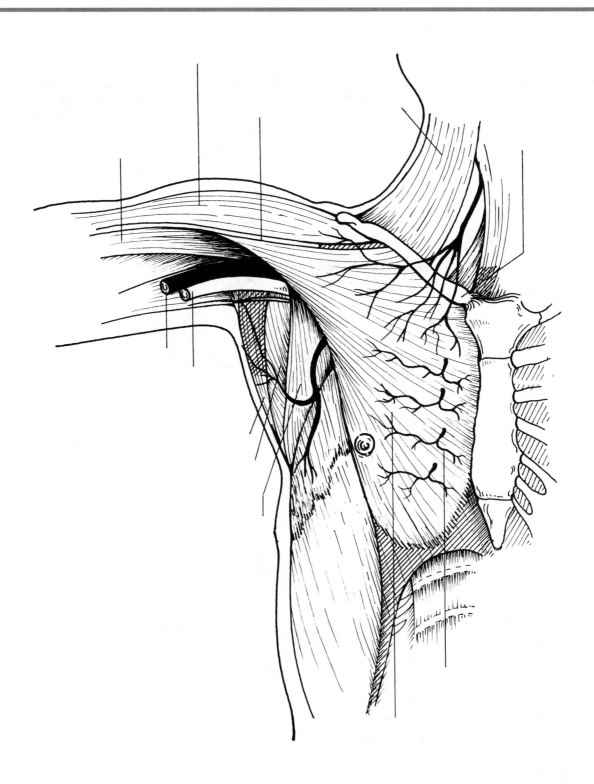

Anterior cutaneous branch of intercostal nerve	Cephalic vein	Pectoralis major
Axillary artery	Deltoid	Subscapularis
Axillary vein	Latissimus dorsi	Teres major
Biceps	Medial end of clavicle	Trapezius

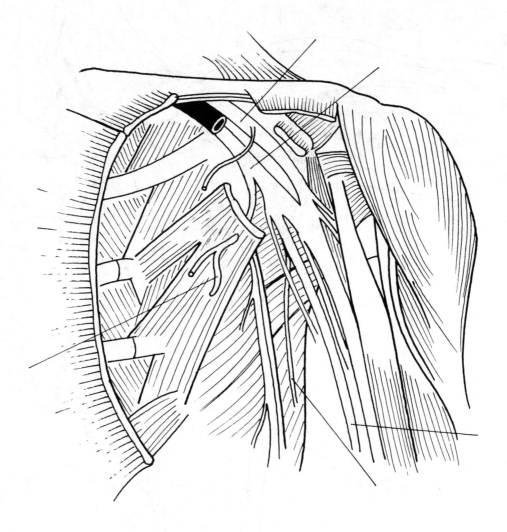

Lateral cord of brachial plexus

Medial cord of brachial plexus

Medial pectoral nerve

Thoracodorsal nerve

Ulnar nerve

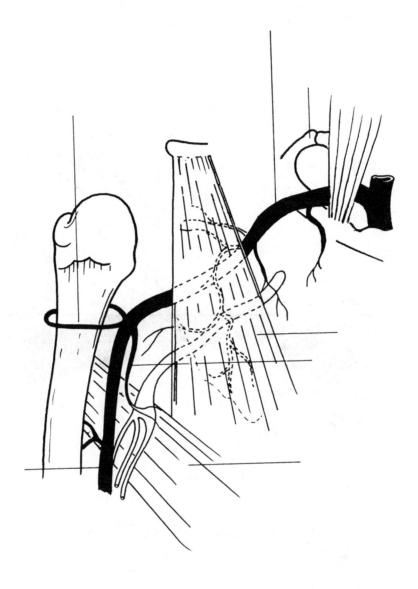

1st rib

Axillary artery

Brachial artery

Circumflex humeral arteries

Lateral thoracic artery

Pectoralis minor

Teres major

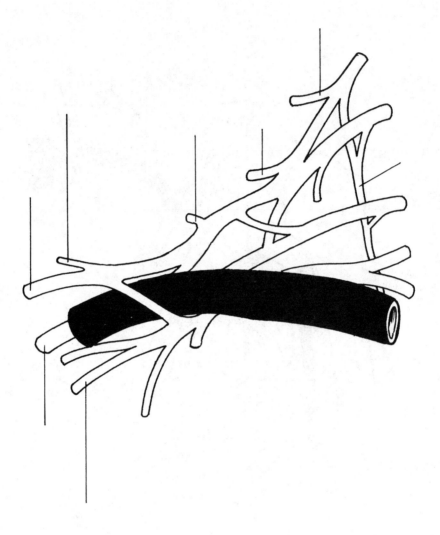

Dorsal scapular nerve   Musculocutaneous nerve

Lateral pectoral nerve   Radial nerve

Long thoracic nerve   Suprascapular nerve

Median nerve   Ulnar nerve

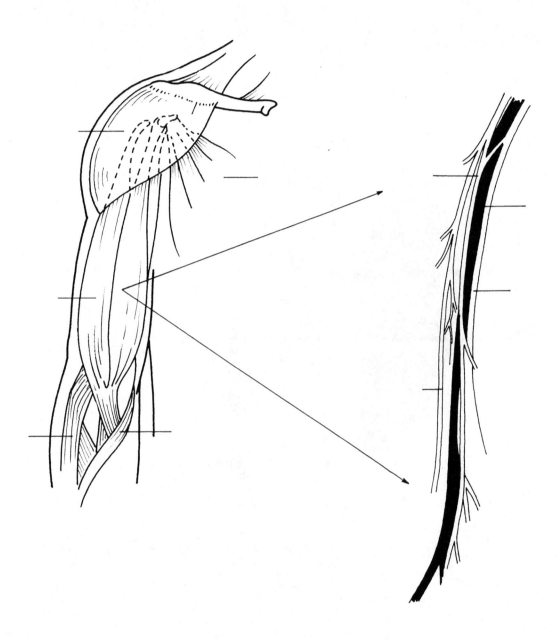

Biceps muscle

Brachial artery

Brachioradialis

Deltoid muscle

Median nerve

Musculocutaneous nerve

Pectoralis minor

Pronator teres

Ulnar nerve

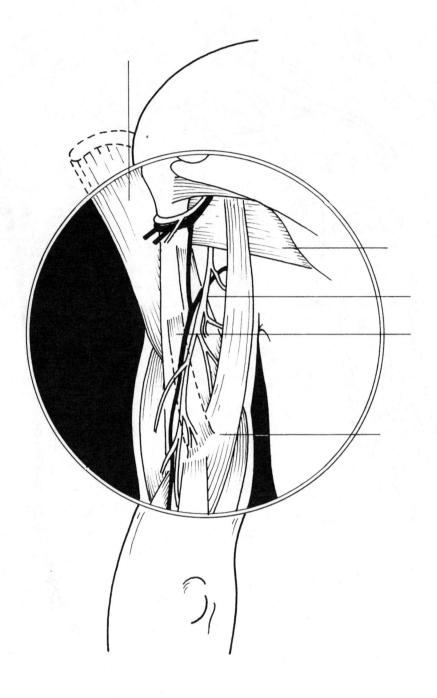

Deltoid

Long head of triceps

Medial head of triceps

Radial nerve

Teres major

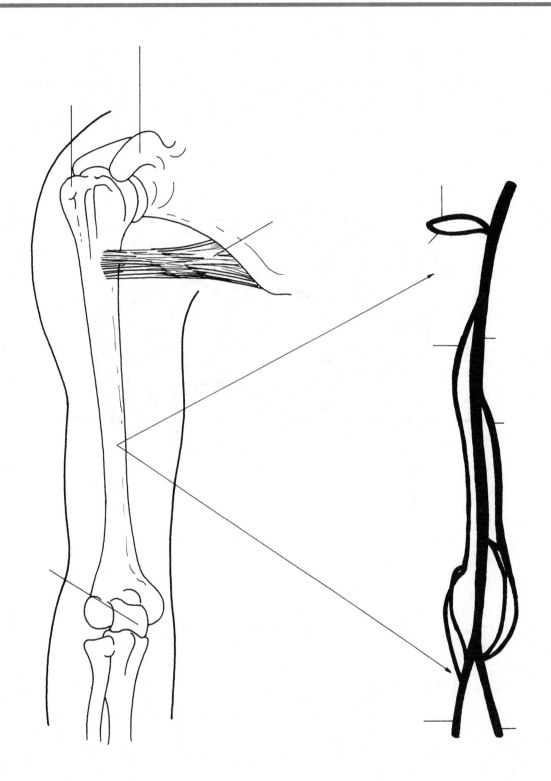

Anterior humeral circumflex
artery

Brachial artery

Coracoid process

Greater tuberosity of humerus

Posterior humeral circumflex
artery

Profunda brachii artery

Radial artery

Superior ulnar collateral artery

Teres major

Trochlea

Ulnar artery

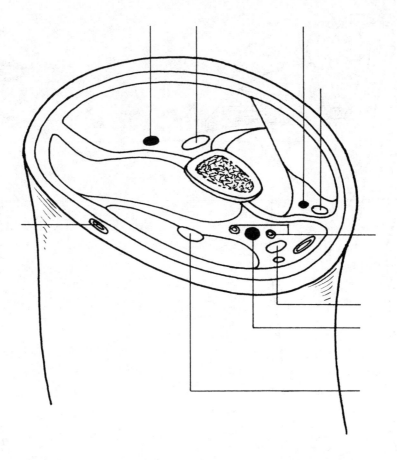

Brachial artery

Cephalic vein

Median nerve

Musculocutaneous nerve

Profunda brachii artery

Radial nerve

Superior ulnar artery

Ulnar nerve

Venae comitantes

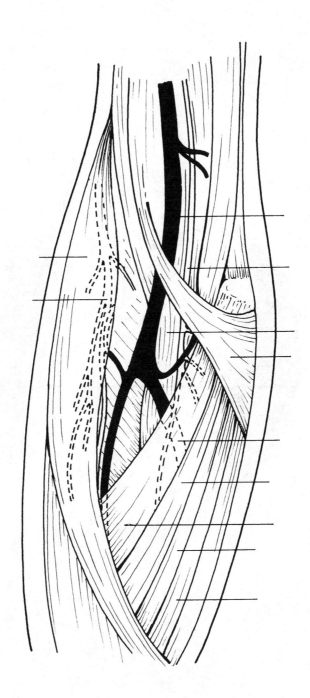

Biceps tendon

Bicipital aponeurosis

Brachial artery

Brachioradialis

Flexor carpi radialis

Flexor carpi ulnaris

Humeral head of pronator teres

Median nerve

Palmaris longus

Radial nerve

Ulnar artery

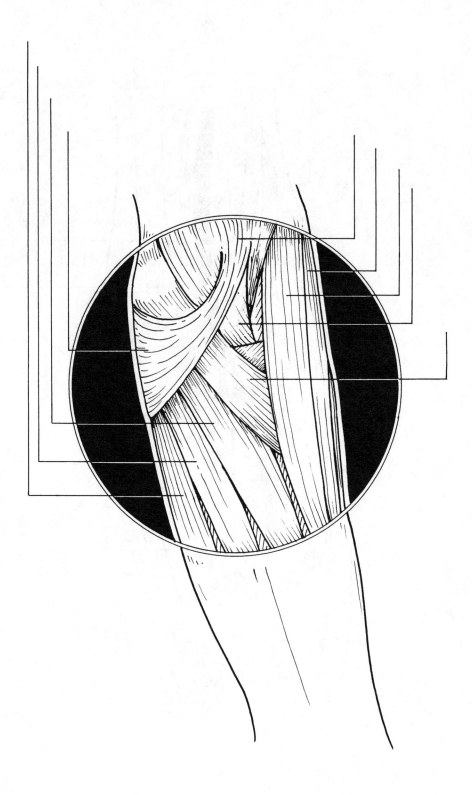

Biceps brachii

Biceps tendon

Bicipital aponeurosis

Brachioradialis

Extensor carpi radialis longus

Flexor carpi radialis

Flexor carpi ulnaris

Palmaris longus

Pronator teres

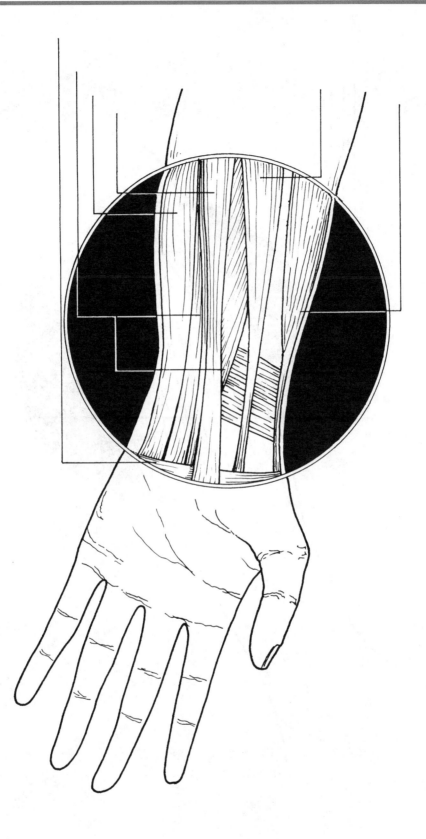

Brachioradialis

Flexor carpi radialis

Flexor carpi ulnaris

Flexor digitorum superficialis

Flexor retinaculum

Palmaris longus

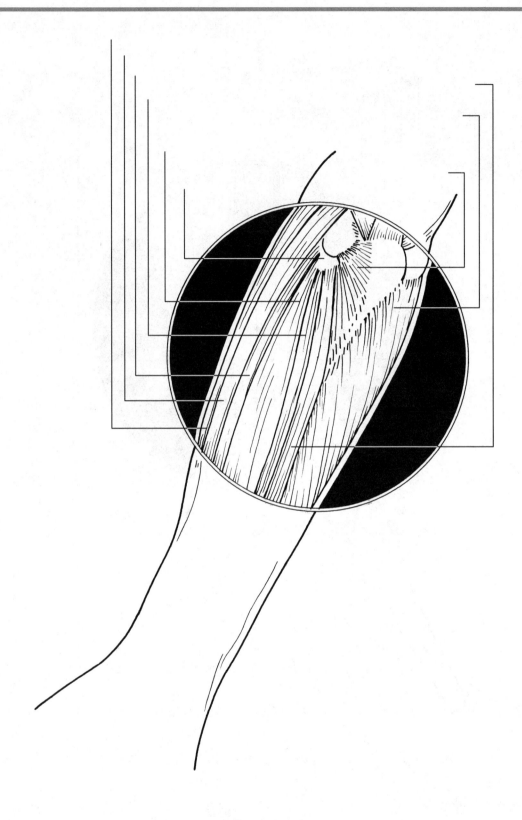

Anconeus

Brachioradialis

Common extensor origin

Extensor carpi radialis brevis

Extensor carpi radialis longus

Extensor carpi ulnaris

Extensor digiti minimi

Extensor digitorum

Flexor carpi ulnaris

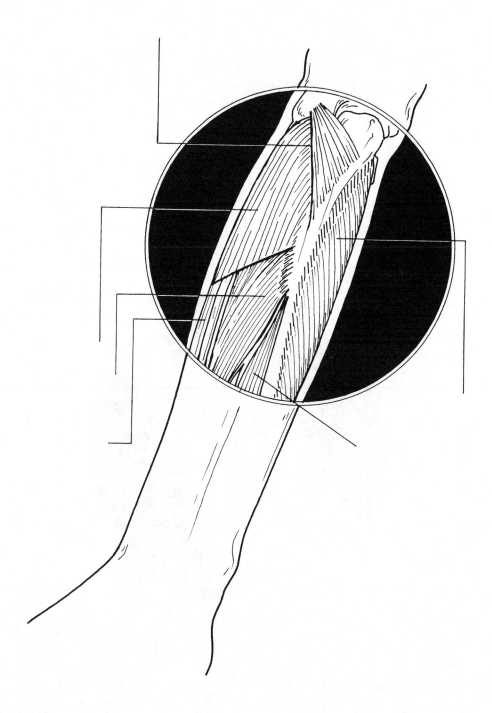

Abductor pollicis longus

Anconeus

Extensor indicis

Extensor pollicis longus

Flexor carpi ulnaris

Supinator

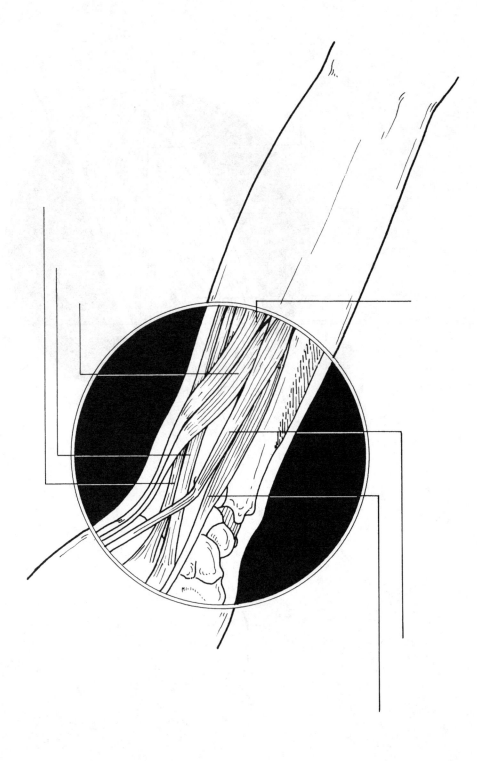

Abductor pollicis longus

Extensor carpi radialis brevis

Extensor carpi radialis longus

Extensor indicis

Extensor pollicis brevis

Extensor pollicis longus

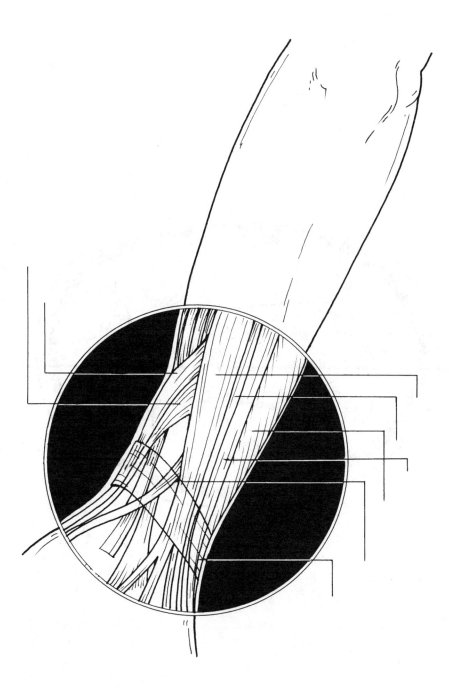

Abductor pollicis longus

Extensor carpi ulnaris

Extensor digiti minimi

Extensor digitorum

Extensor pollicis brevis

Extensor pollicis longus

Extensor retinaculum

Flexor carpi ulnaris

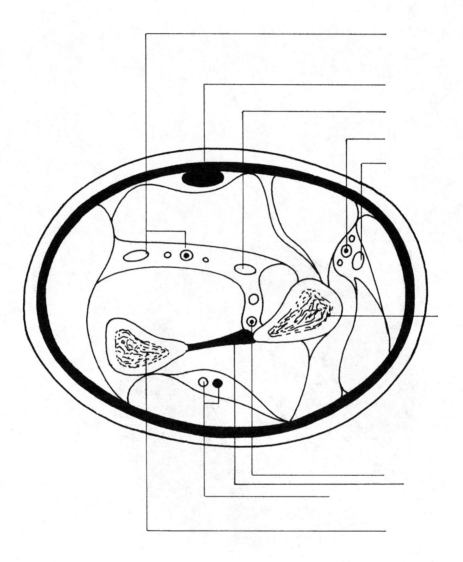

Anterior interosseous artery

Interosseus membrane

Median nerve

Palmaris longus

Posterior interosseous nerve and
artery

Radial artery

Radial nerve (superficial branch)

Radius

Ulna

Ulnar nerve and artery

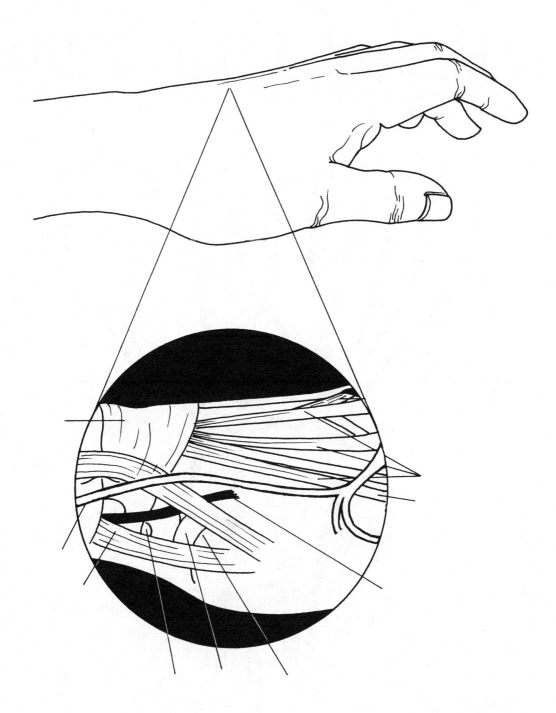

Base of first metacarpal

Cephalic vein

Extensor pollicis brevis

Extensor retinaculum

Radial artery

Scaphoid

Styloid process of radius

Tendon of extensor digitorum

Tendon of extensor indicis

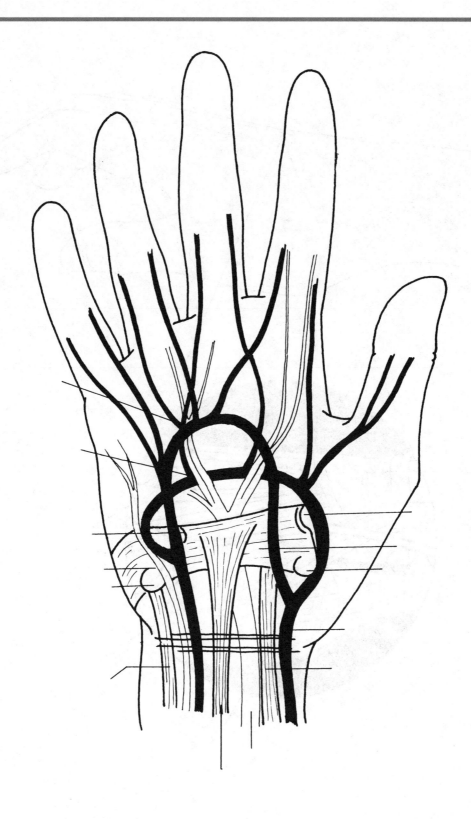

Deep palmar arch	Median nerve	Scaphoid
Flexor carpi radialis	Palmaris longus	Superficial palmar arch
Flexor carpi ulnaris	Pisiform	Ulnar nerve
Flexor retinaculum	Radial artery	
Hook of hamate	Ridge of trapezium	

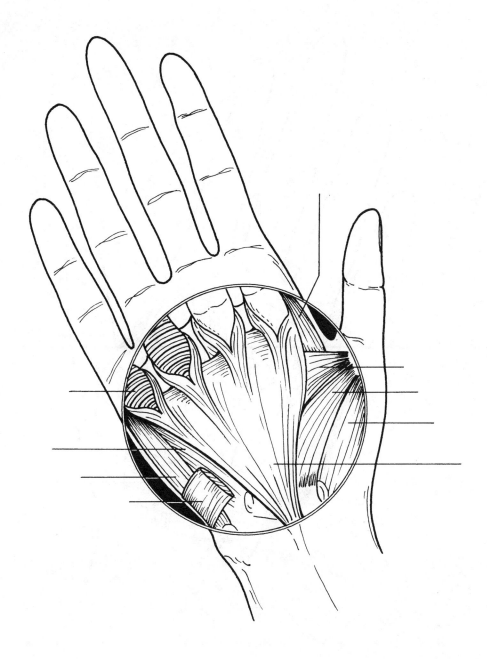

1st dorsal interosseous

Abductor digiti minimi

Abductor pollicis brevis

Adductor pollicis

Flexor digiti minimi

Flexor pollicis brevis

Fibrous flexor sheath

Palmar aponeurosis

Palmaris brevis

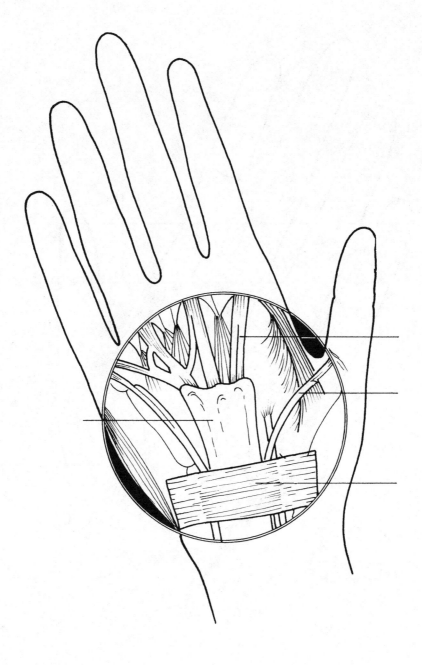

Extensor indicis

Extensor retinaculum

Synovial sheath

Tendon of flexor pollicis longus

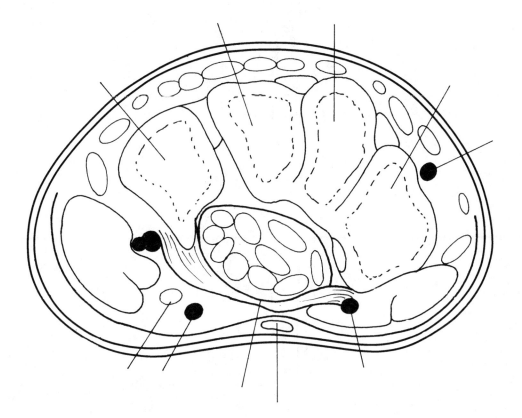

Capitate	Superficial palmar artery
Flexor retinaculum	Trapezium
Hamate	Trapezoid
Palmaris longus	Ulnar artery
Radial artery	Ulnar nerve

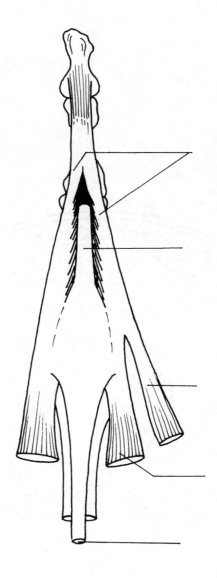

Central slip of extensor
expansion

Extensor digitorum tendon

Interosseous muscle

Lateral slip of extensor expansion

Lumbrical muscle

Section 4
ABDOMEN

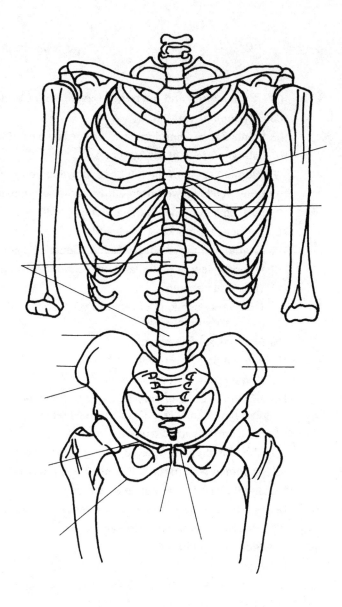

Anterior superior iliac spine

Iliac crest

Iliac fossa

Inguinal ligament

Ischial tuberosity

Lumbar vertebrae

Pubic crest

Symphysis pubis

Tubercle of iliac crest

Xiphisternal joint

Xiphoid process

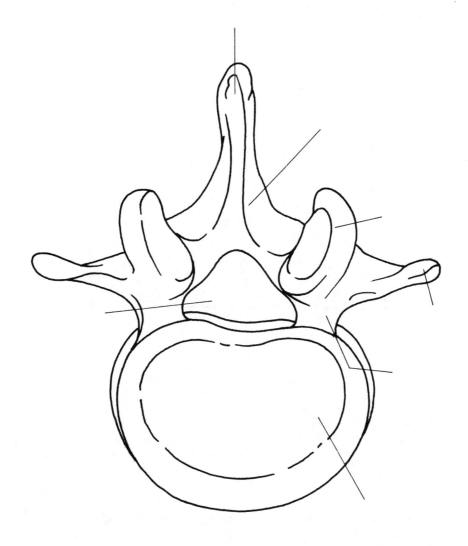

Body   Superior articular process

Lamina   Transverse process

Pedicle   Vertebral canal

Spinous process

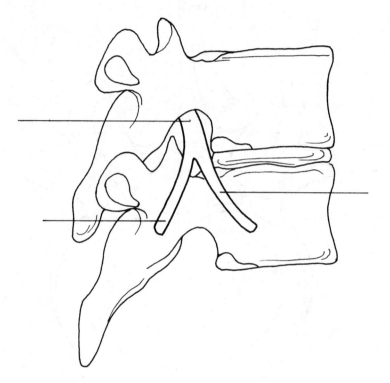

Dorsal ramus

Spinal nerve

Ventral ramus

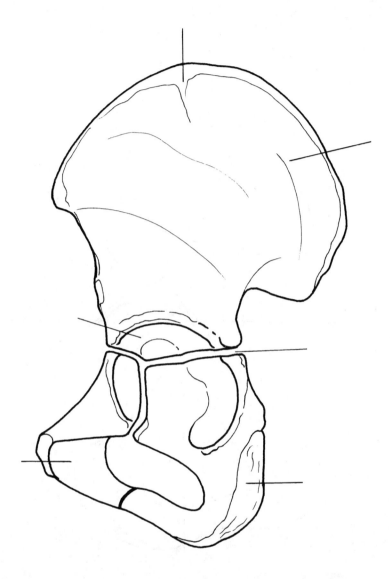

Acetabulum

Ilium

Ischium

Line of fusion of hip bones

Pubis

Tubercle of ilium/iliac crest

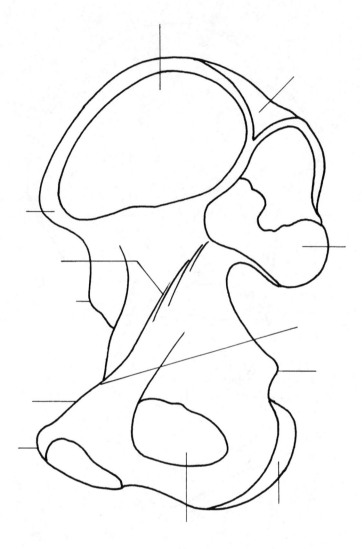

Anterior inbferior iliac spine

Anterior superior iliac spine

Arcuate line

Articular surface for sacrum

Iliacus muscle

Ischial spine

Ischial tuberosity

Obturator foramen

Pectineal line

Pubic crest

Pubic tubercle

Quadratus lumborum muscle

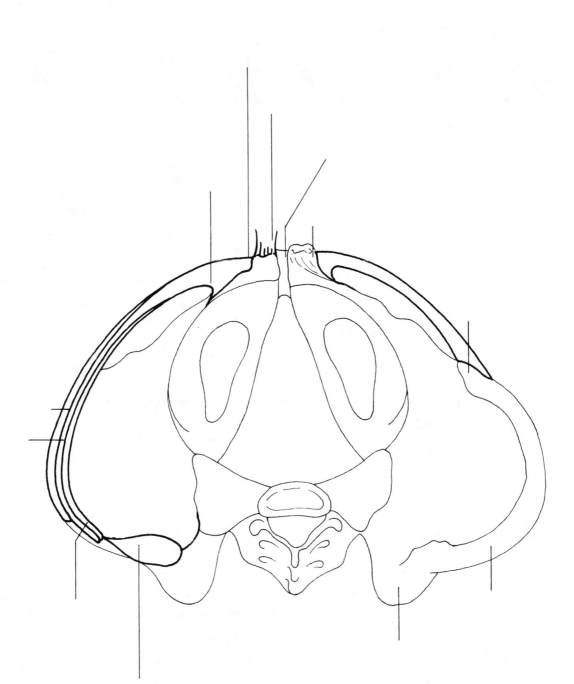

Anterior superior iliac spine

Attachment of external oblique

Attachment of internal oblique

Attachment of quadratus
lumborum

Attachment of transversus
abdominis

Inguinal ligament

Lacunar ligament

Pectineal ligament

Posterior superior iliac spine

Pubic tubercle

Rectus abdominis (reflected
anteriorly)

Symphysis pubis

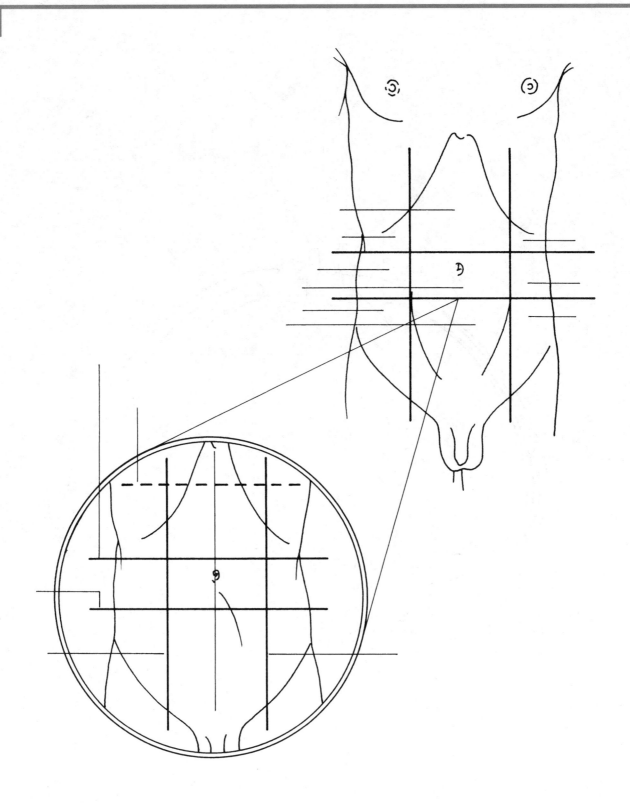

Epigastrium

Hypogastrium

Intertubercular (transtubercular) plane

Left hypochondrium

Left iliac region

Left lumbar region

Left vertical line (plane)

Right hypochondrium

Right iliac region

Right lumbar region

Right vertical line (plane)

Subcostal plane

Transpyloric plane

Umbilical region

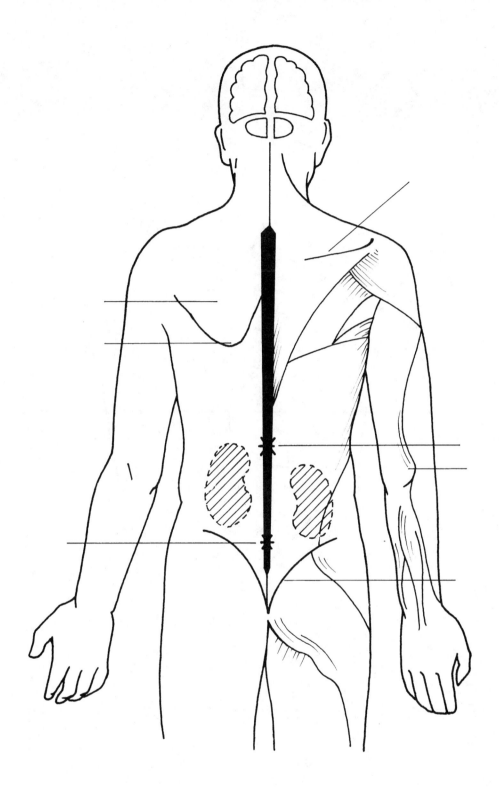

Angle of scapula

Iliac crest

Lateral epicondyle of humerus

Scapula

Spine of scapula

Spinous process of L3

Spinous process of T12

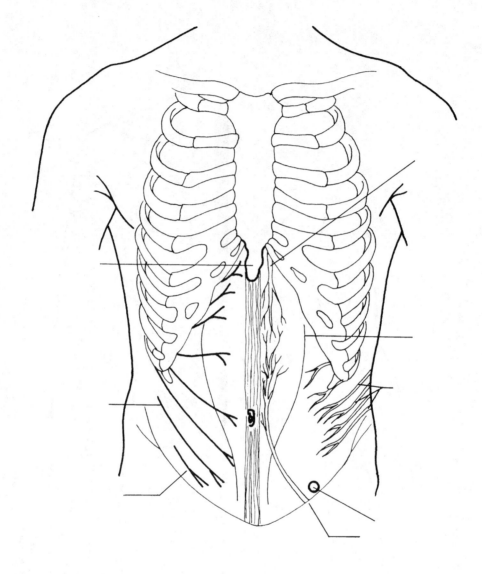

Deep inguinal ring

Iliohypogastric nerve

Ilioinguinal nerve

Inferior epigastric artery

Lateral margin of rectus sheath

Lumbar arteries

Superior epigastric artery

Xiphoid process

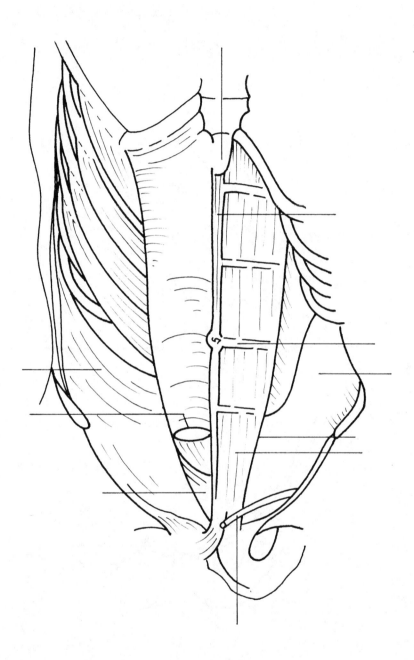

Arcuate line	Pyramidalis
External oblique	Rectus abdominis
Internal oblique muscle	Spermatic cord
Linea alba	Tendinous intersections
Linea semilunaris	Xiphoid process

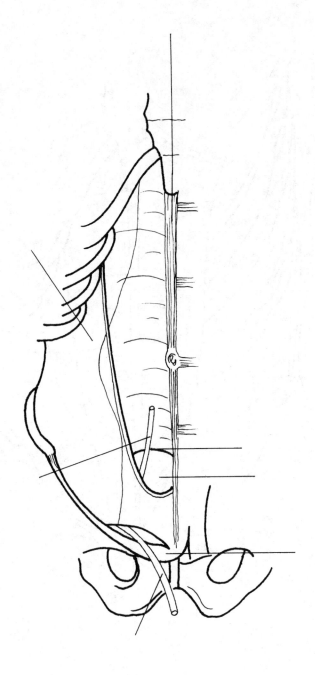

Arcuate line

Conjoint tendon

Fascia transversalis

Inferior epigastric artery

Linea alba

Spermatic cord

Transversus abdominis

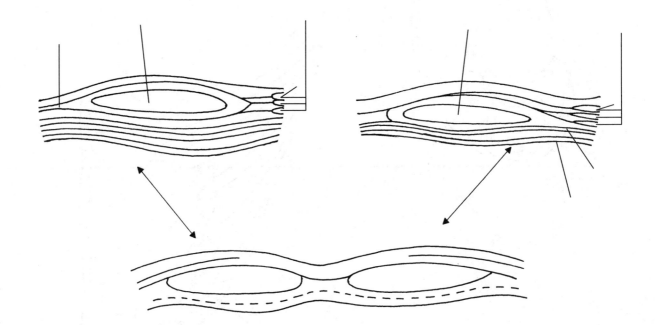

External oblique

Internal oblique

Linea alba

Peritoneum

Rectus abdominis

Transversalis fascia

Transversus abdominis

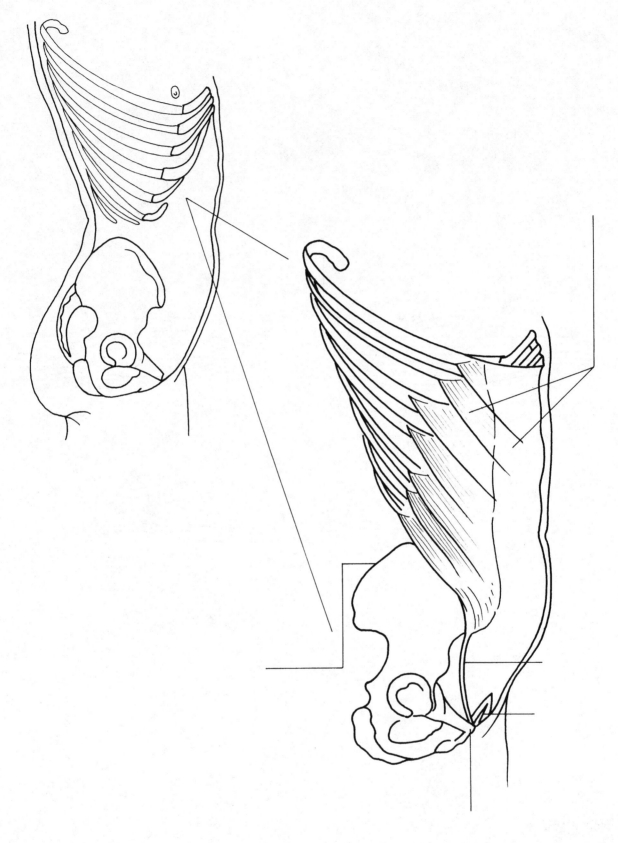

External oblique

Iliac crest

Inguinal ligament

Pubic tubercle

Superficial inguinal ring

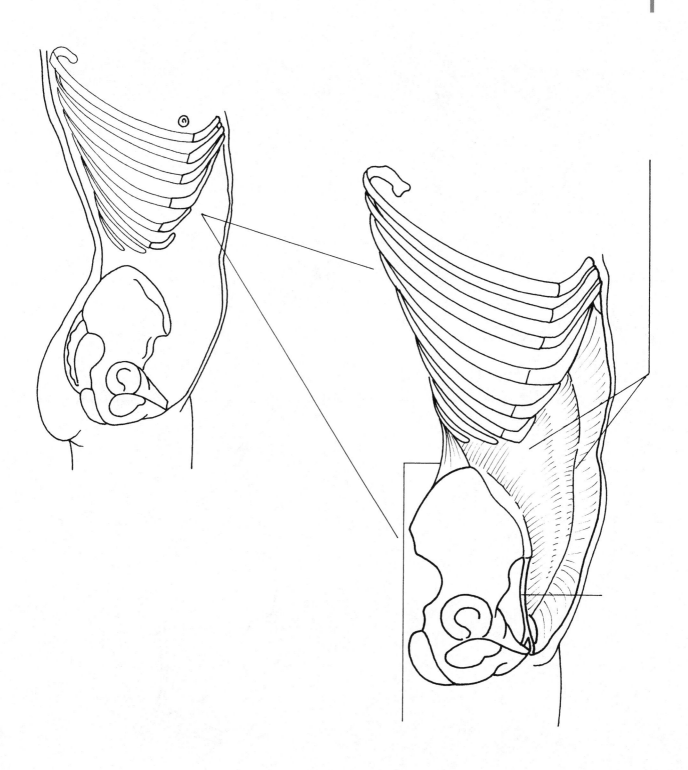

Inguinal ligament

Internal oblique

Lumbar fascia

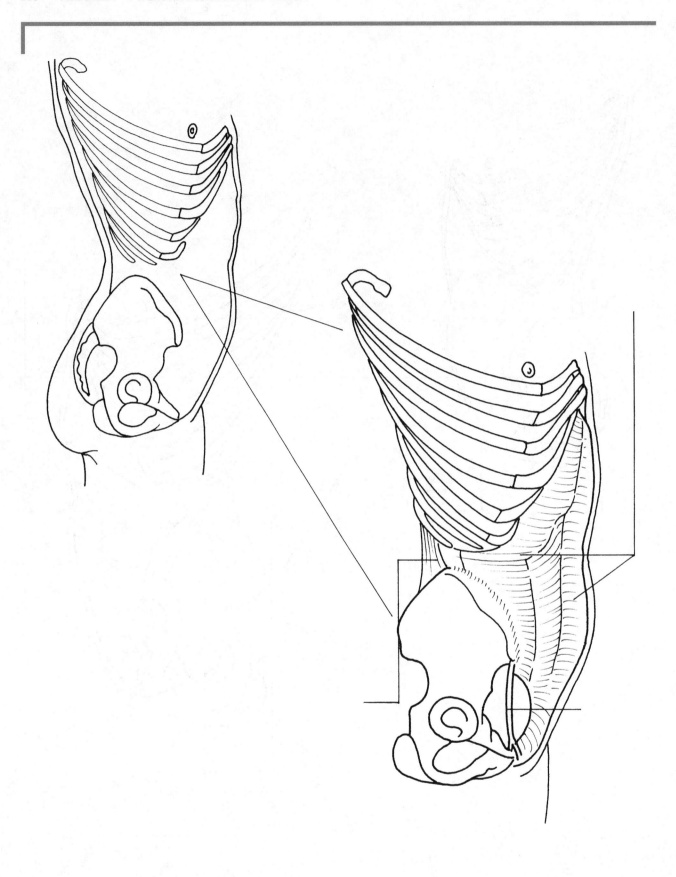

Inguinal ligament

Lumbar fascia

Transversus abdominis

A

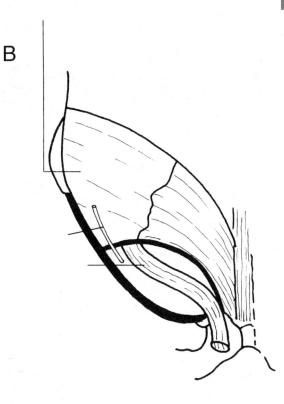

B

C

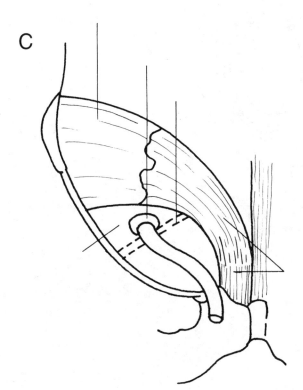

D

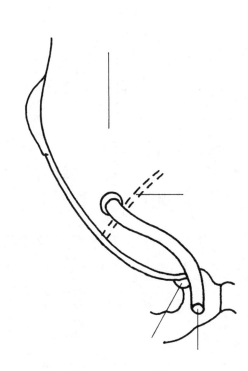

Conjoint tendon

Cremaster muscle

Deep inguinal ring

Fascia transversalis

Ilioinguinal nerve

Inferior epigastric artery

Internal oblique

Linea alba

Spermatic cord

Superficial inguinal ring

Transversus abdominis

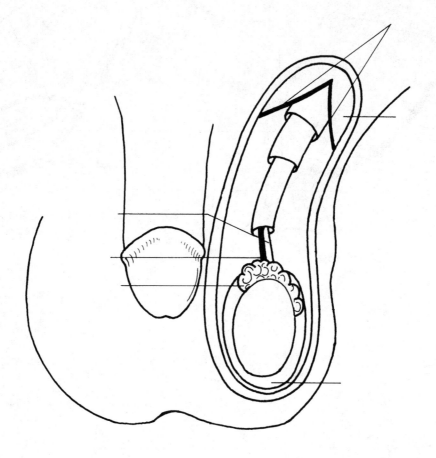

Aponeurosis of external oblique

Epidydimis

Superficial inguinal ring

Testicular artery

Tunica vaginalis

Vas deference

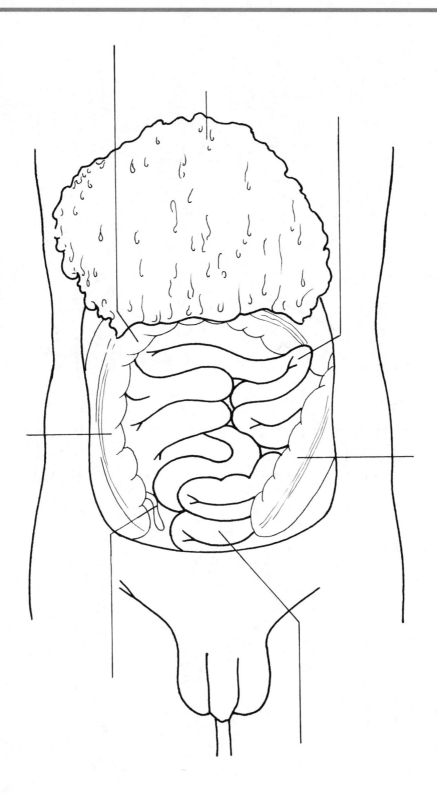

Appendix

Ascending colon

Coils of small intestine

Descending colon

Greater omentum

Transverse colon

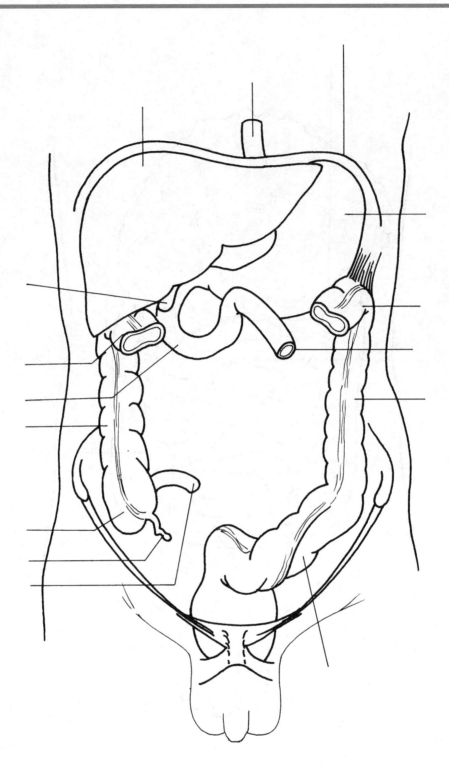

Appendix

Ascending colon

Cecum

Descending colon

Duodenum

Gallbladder

Ileum

Jejunum

Left colic flexure

Left dome of diaphragm

Liver

Oesophagus

Right colic flexure

Sigmoid colon

Stomach

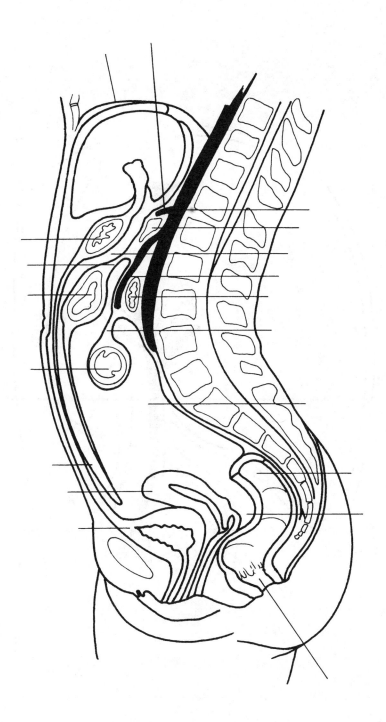

Anal canal

Aorta

Bladder

Coeliac artery

Diaphragm

Greater omentum

Greater sac

Lesser omentum

Lesser sac

Mesentery

Pancreas

Rectouterine pouch

Rectum

Stomach

Superior mesenteric artery

Third part of duodenum

Transverse colon

Transverse mesocolon

Uterus

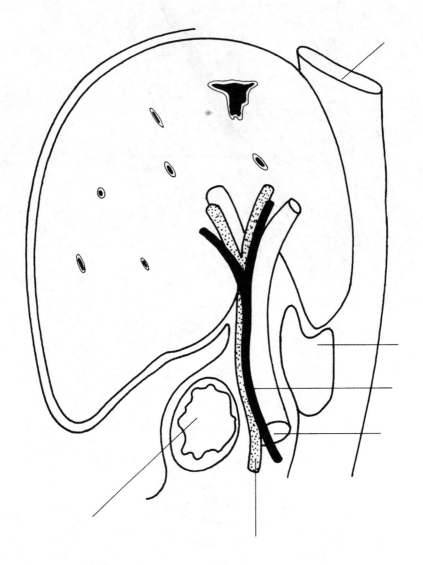

Common bile duct

Duodenum

Epiploic foramen

Hepatic artery

Inferior vena cava

Portal vein

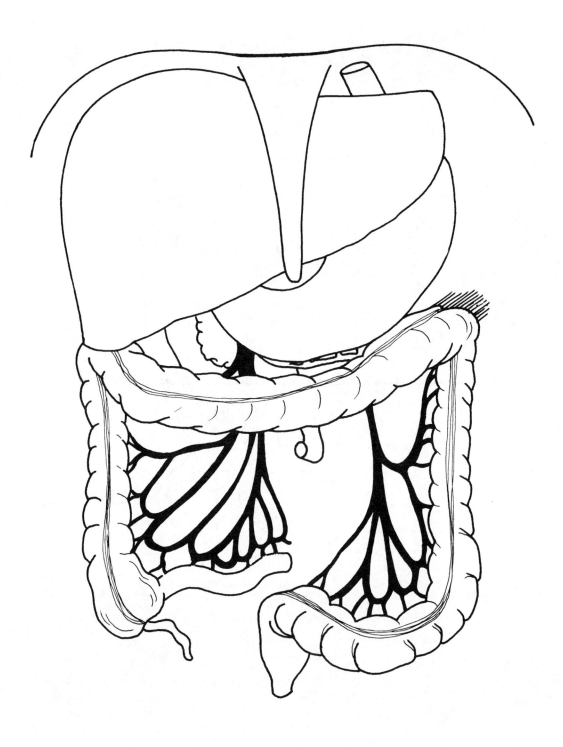

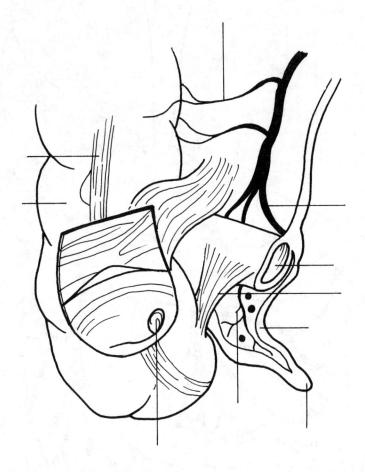

Appendicular artery

Appendix

Ascending colon

Caecal branches of ileocaecal artery

Ileal branches of ileocaecal artery

Ileocaecal fold

Ileum

Mesentery of appendix

Opening of appendix

Taenia coli

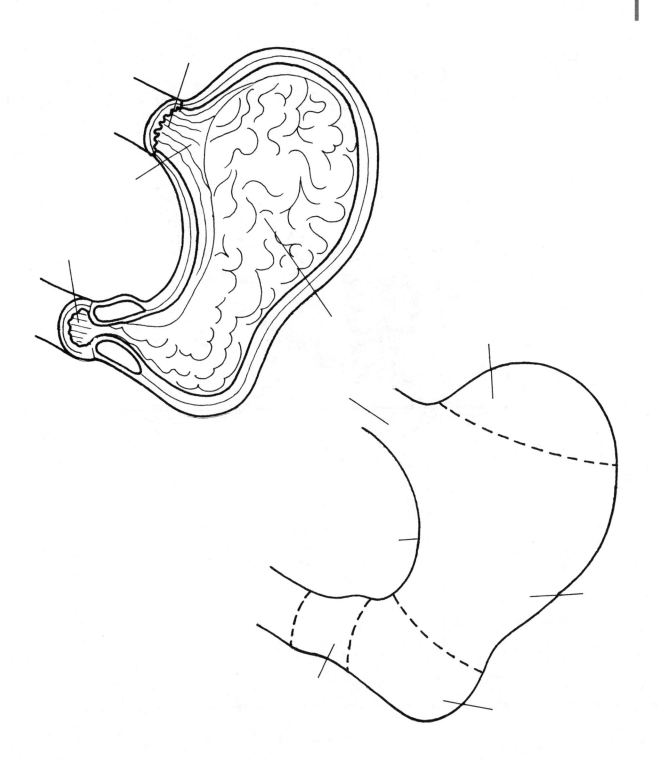

Antrum	Lesser curvature
Body	Longitudinal folds of mucous coat
Cardiac orifice	Oesophagus
Fundus	Pyloric sphincter
Greater curvature	Pyloris

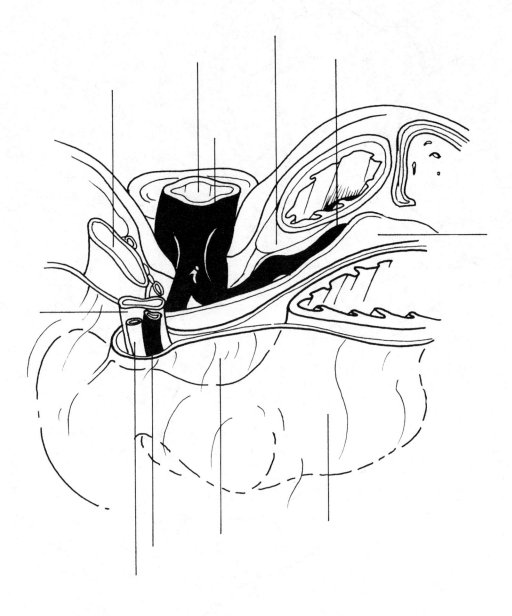

Abdominal aorta

Coeliac artery

Common bile duct

Hepatic artery

Inferior vena cava

Left suprarenal gland

Lesser omentum

Lesser sac

Outline of stomach

Portal vein

Splenic artery

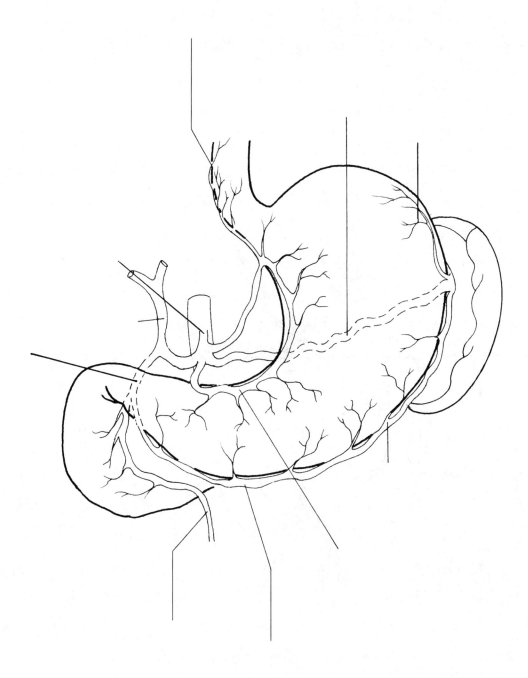

Coeliac trunk	Right gastric artery
Gastroduodenal artery	Right gastroepiploic artery
Hepatic artery	Short gastric arteries
Left gastroepiploic artery	Splenic artery
Oesophageal branches	Superior pancreaticoduodenal artery

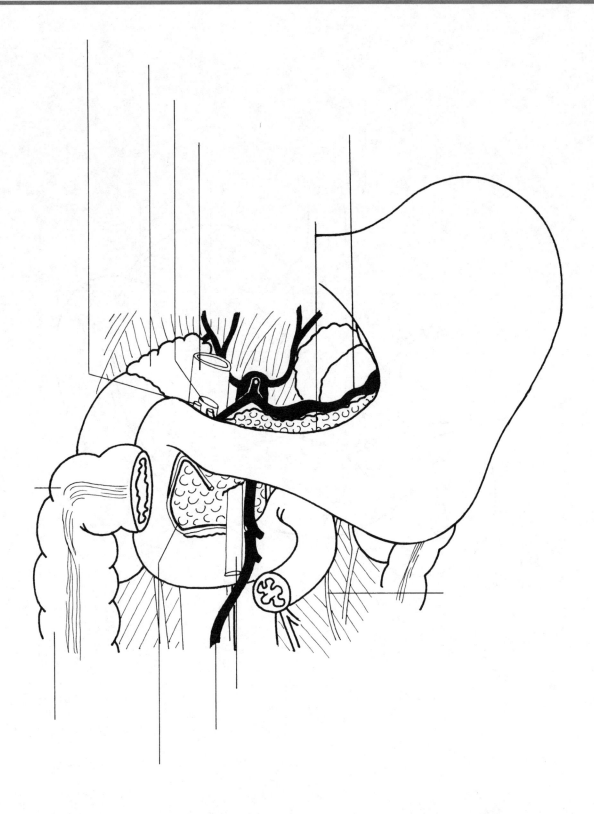

Ascending colon	Right colic flexure
Common bile duct	Right suprarenal gland
Inferior mesenteric vein	Splenic artery
Inferior vena cava	Superior mesenteric artery
Pancreas	Superior mesenteric vein
Portal vein	Tail of pancreas

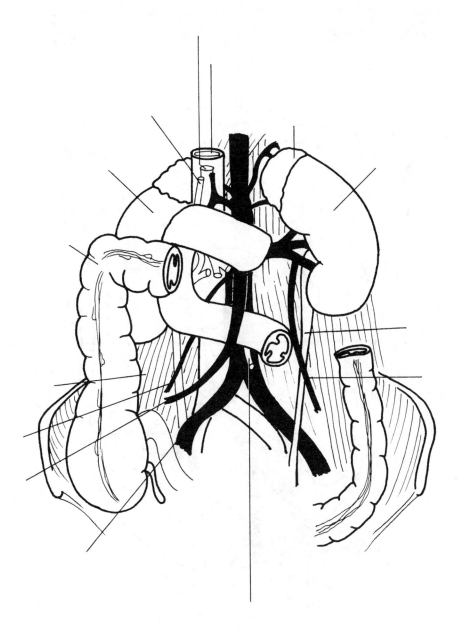

Common bile duct

Inferior mesenteric artery (in white)

Inferior vena cava

Left kidney

Left gonadal vein (in black)

Left suprarenal gland

Left ureter

Portal vein

Psoas major

Right colic flexure

Right common iliac artery

Right kidney

Right testicular artery

Superior mesenteric artery

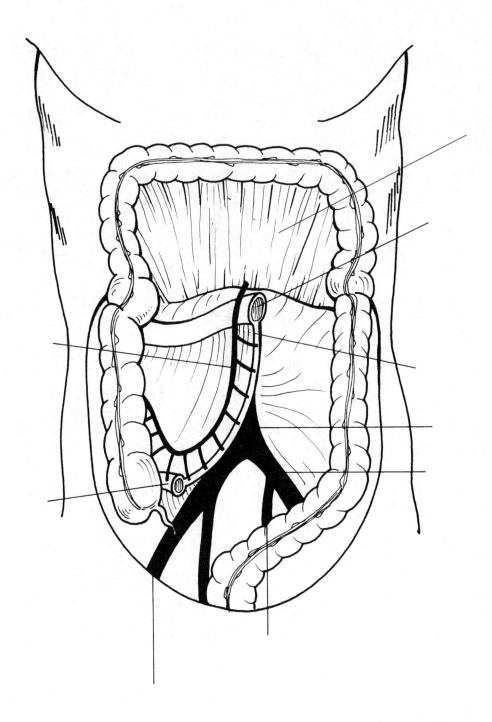

Abdominal aorta

Duodenojejunal junction

External iliac artery

Ileocolic junction

Internal iliac artery

Left common iliac artery

Root of mesentery of small intestine

Superior mesenteric artery

Transverse mesocolon

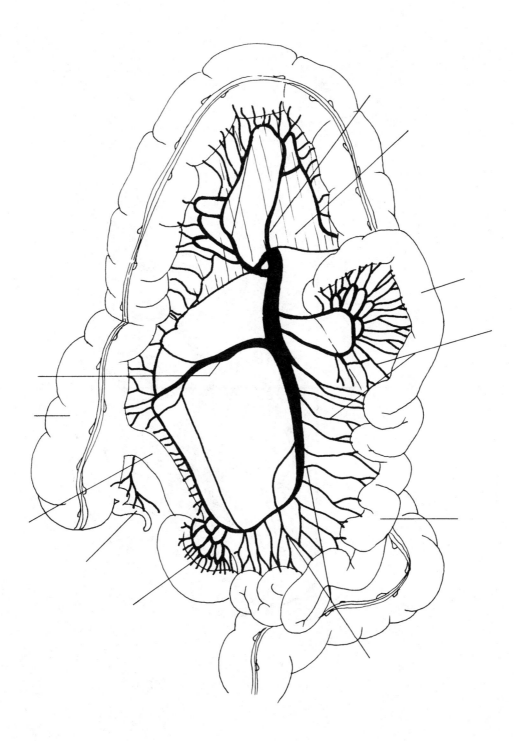

Appendix

Arterial arcades

Ascending colon

Ileal arteries

Ileocolic artery

Ileum

Jejunal arteries

Jejunum

Middle colic artery

Transverse mesocolon

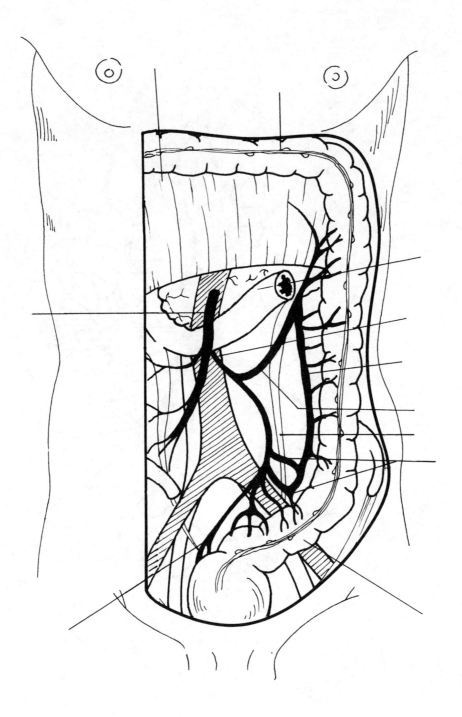

Duodenum

Inferior mesenteric artery

Left colic artery

Left ureter

Marginal artery

Omentum

Rectal artery

Sigmoid arteries

Sigmoid colon

Superior mesenteric artery

Transverse colon

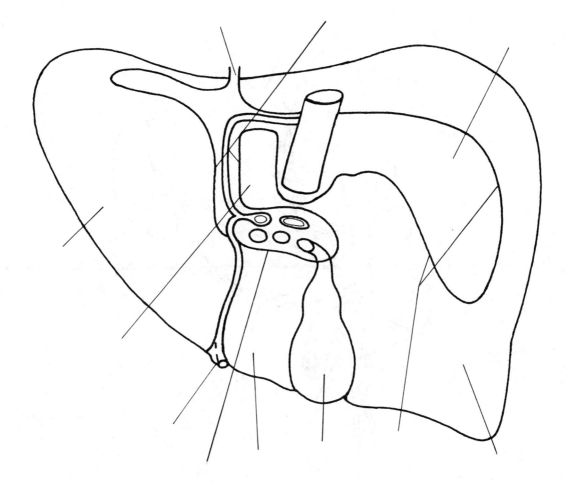

Bare area

Caudate lobe

Coronary ligament

Falciform ligament

Fissure for ligamentum venosum

Gallbladder

Left lobe

Ligamentum teres

Porta hepatis

Quadrate lobe

Right lobe

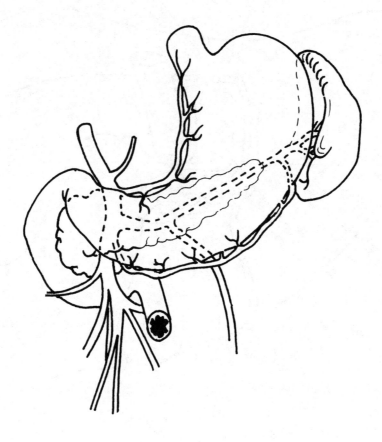

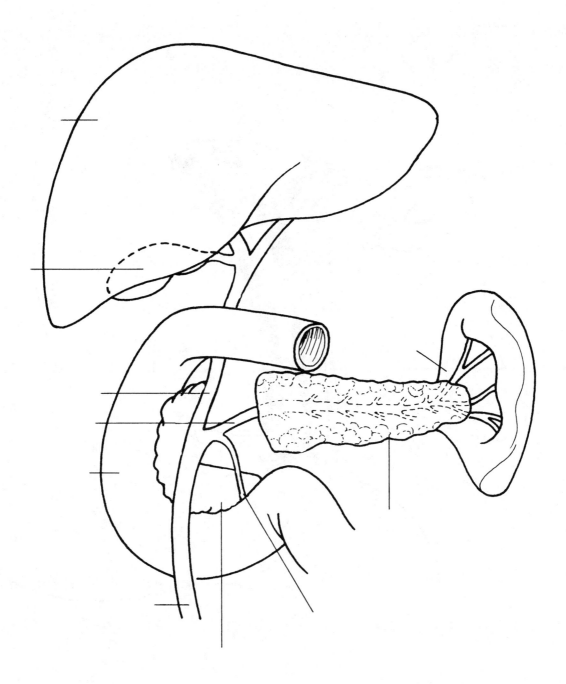

2nd part of duodenum	Liver
Body of pancreas	Portal vein
Gallbladder	Spleen
Uncinate process of pancreas	Splenic vein
Inferior mesenteric vein	Superior mesenteric vein

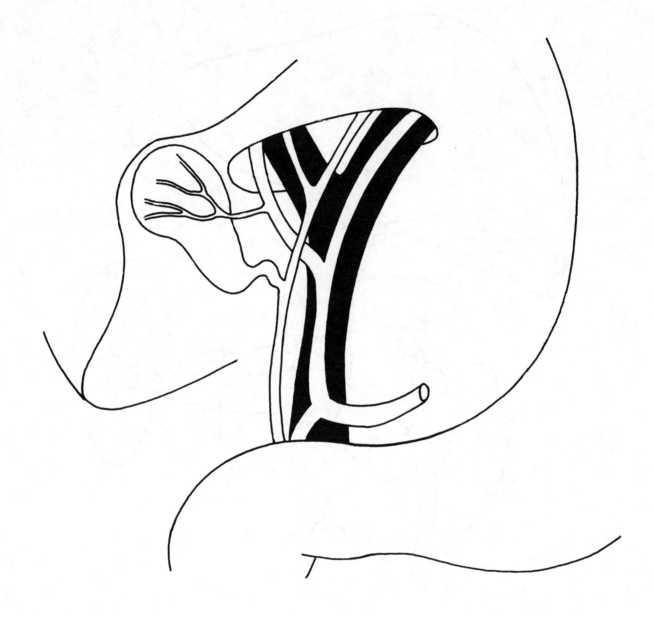

(Veins black, arteries white)

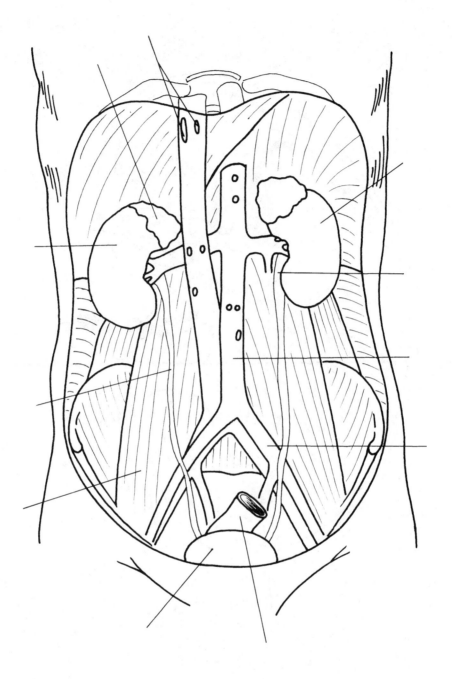

Abdominal aorta

Hepatic veins

Left common iliac artery

Left kidney

Pelvis of ureter

Psoas major

Rectum

Right kidney

Right suprarenal gland

Right ureter

Urinary bladder

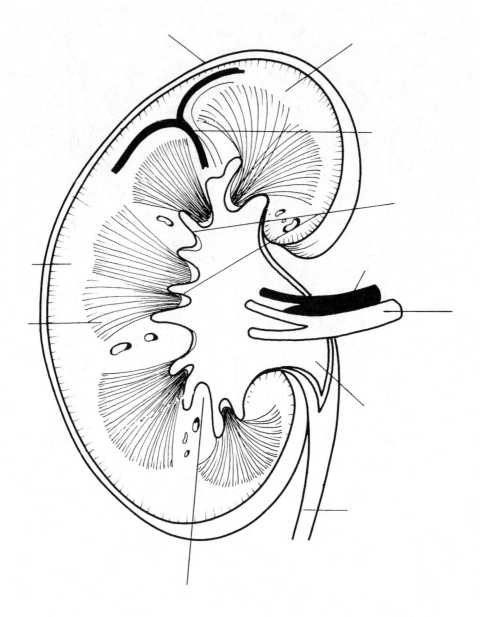

Capsule	Pyramid
Cortex	Renal artery
Interlobar artery and vein	Renal papilla
Major calyx	Renal vein
Minor calyces	Ureter

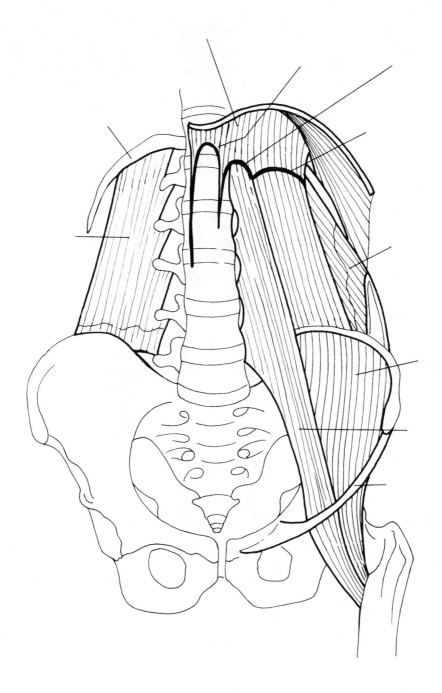

12th rib	Medial arcuate ligament
Iliacus	Median arcuate ligament
Inguinal ligament	Psoas major
Lateral arcuate ligament	Quadratus lumborum
Left dome of diaphragm	Transversus abdominis

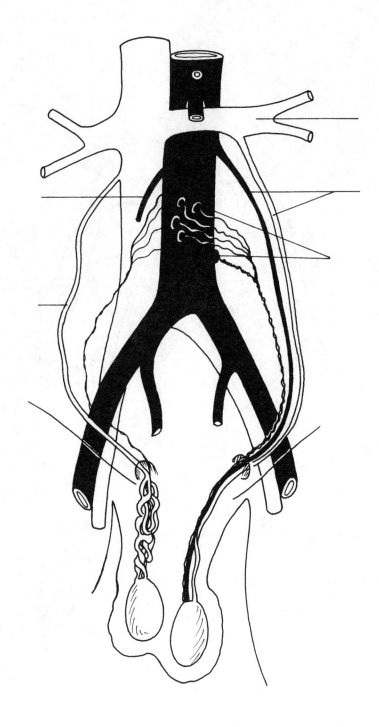

Left renal vein

Left testicular vessels

Para-aortic lymph nodes

Right testicular artery

Right testicular vein

Section 5
PELVIS AND PERINEUM

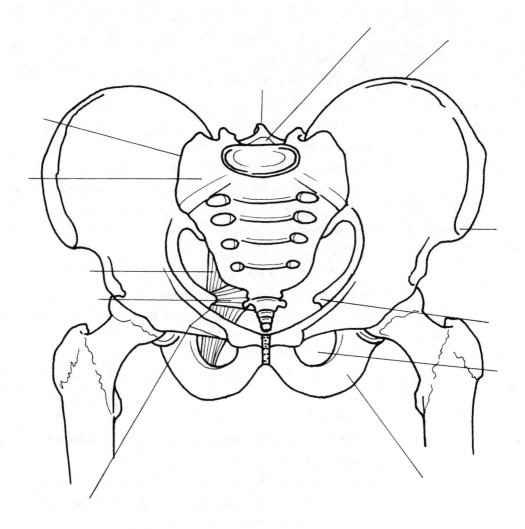

Anterior superior iliac spine

First sacral spine

Iliac crest

Ischial spine

Lateral mass of sacrum

Obturator foramen

Pubic crest

Ramus of ischium

Sacral canal

Sacro-iliac joint

Sacrospinous ligament

Sacrotuberous ligament

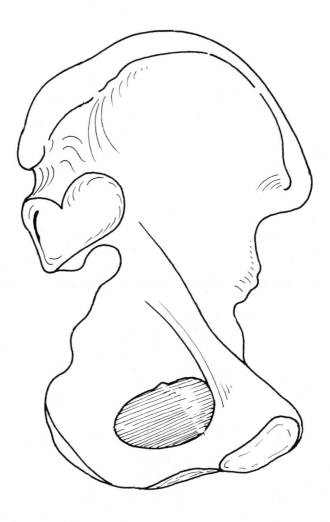

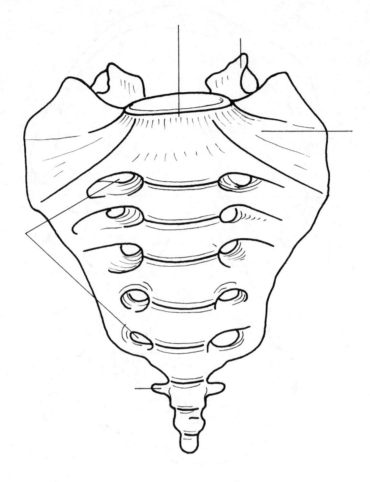

Anterior sacral foramina

Lateral mass

Promontory of sacrum

Superior articular process

Transverse process of coccyx

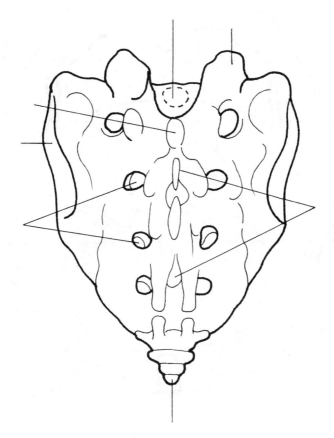

Auricular surface

Sacral canal

First sacral spine

Superior articular process

Median crest

Tip of coccyx

Posterior sacral foramina

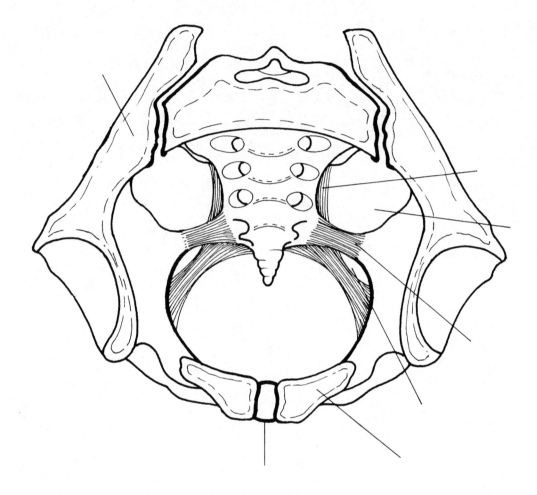

Body of pubis (cut)

Greater sciatic foramen

Ilium

Lesser sciatic foramen

Sacrospinus ligament

Sacrotuberous ligament

Symphysis pubis

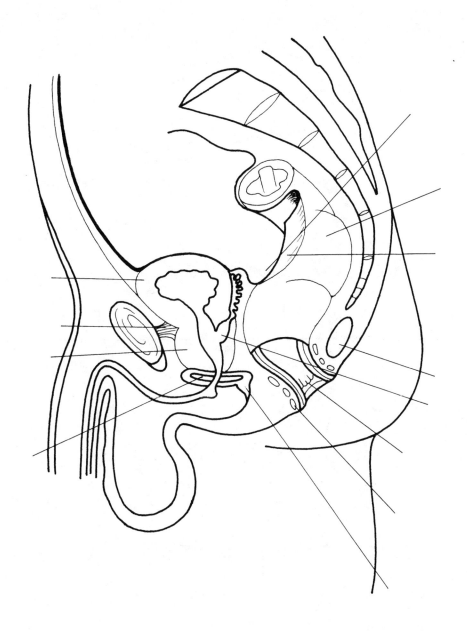

Anal canal	External sphincter	Puboprostatic ligament
Anococcygeal body	Perineal body	Rectovesical pouch
Bladder	Peritoneum	Sigmoid colon
Ejaculatory duct into urethra	Prostate	Urogenital diaphragm

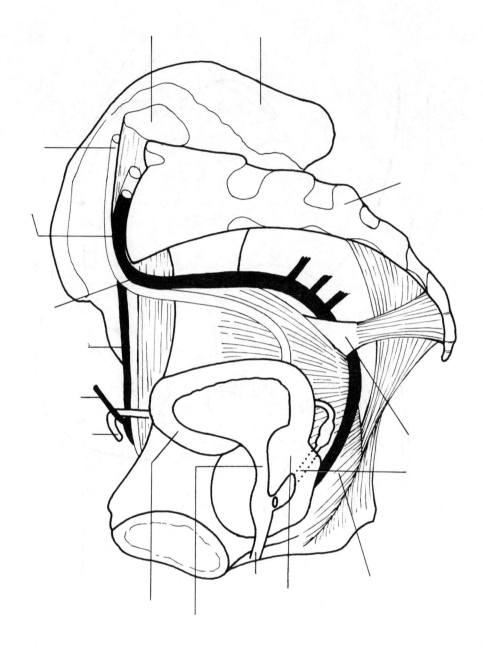

Bladder	Inferior epigastric artery	Prostatic urethra
Common iliac artery	Internal iliac artery	Psoas major (cut)
Ejaculatory duct	Ischial spine	Sacrum
External iliac artery	Obturator internus	Ureter
Ilium	Prostate	Vas deferens

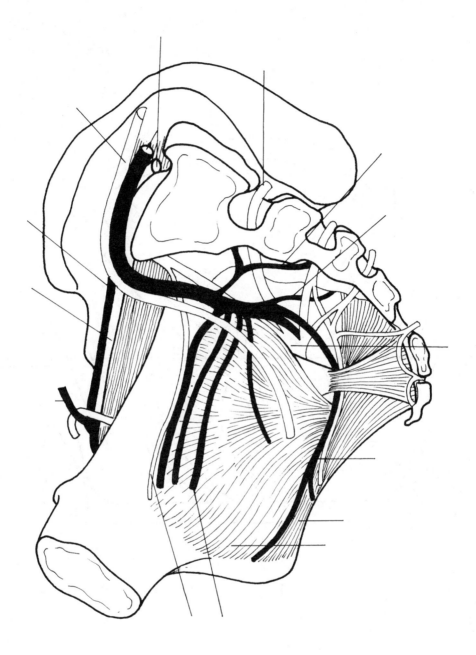

Common iliac artery and vein

External iliac artery

External iliac vein

Inferior epigastric artery

Internal pudendal artery

Lateral sacral artery

Obturator internus muscle

Obturator nerve

S1

Sacrotuberous ligament

Sciatic nerve

Superior gluteal artery

Superior vesicle artery

Ureter

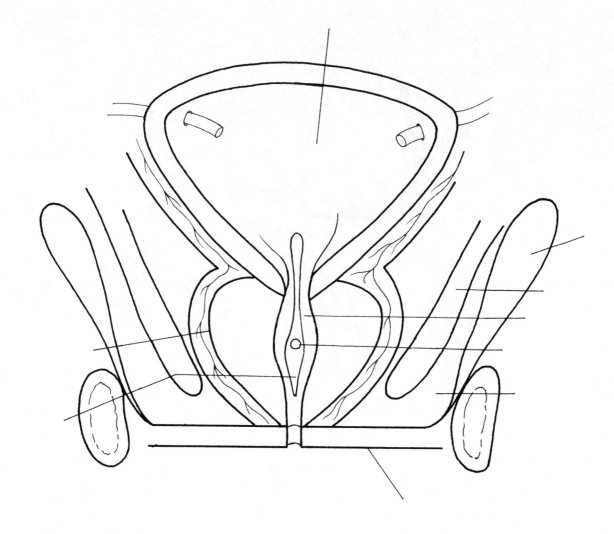

Bladder

Capsule of prostate

Ischiorectal fossa

Levator ani

Mouth of utricle

Obturator internus

Prostatic sinus

Urethral crest

Urogenital diaphragm

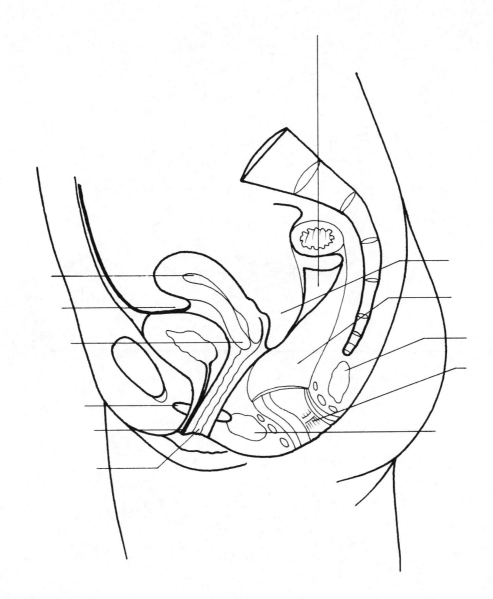

Anal canal	Rectouterine pouch
Anococcygeal body	Rectum
Cavity of uterus	Urethra
Cervix	Urogenital diaphragm
Peritoneum	Uterovesical pouch
Perineal body	Vagina

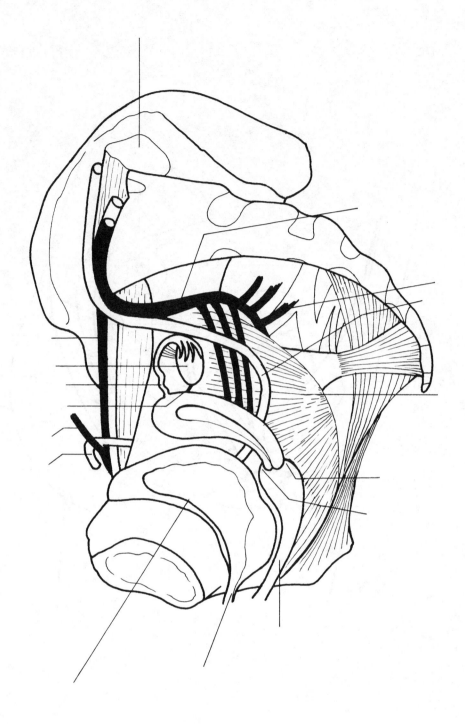

Anterior fornix	Ligament of ovary	Ureter
Bladder	Obturator internus	Urethra
External iliac artery	Ovary	Uterine tube
Inferior epigastric artery	Posterior fornix	Vagina
Inferior gluteal artery	Psoas major (cut)	
Internal iliac artery	Round ligament of uterus	

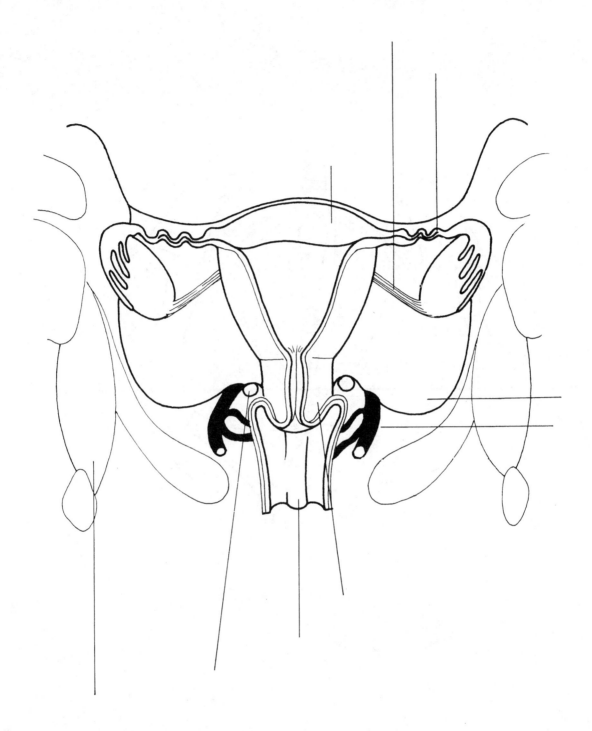

Broad ligament

Cervix

Fundus of uterus

Ligament of ovary

Obturator internus

Ureter

Uterine artery

Uterine tube

Vagina

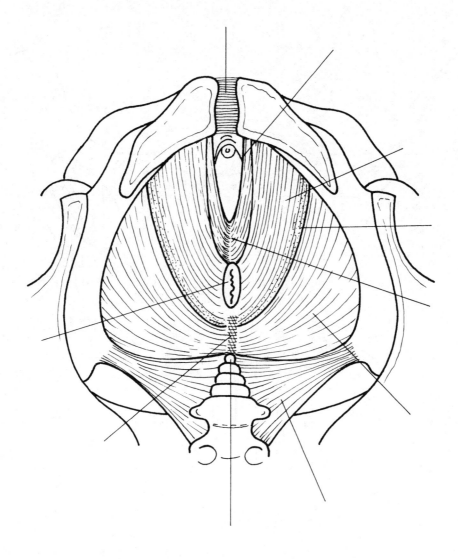

Anococcygeal ligament

Coccygeus

Iliococcygeus

Junction of rectum & anal canal

Levator prostatae/pubovaginalis

Perineal body

Pubococcygeus

Puborectalis

Symphysis pubis

Tip of coccyx

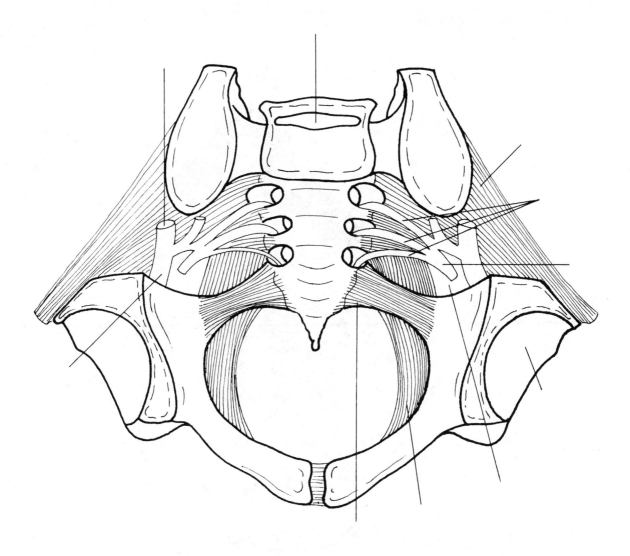

Acetabulum

Anterior rami of sacral spinal
nerves

Greater sciatic foramen

Lumbosacral trunk

Piriformis

Pudendal nerve

Sacral canal

Sacrospinous ligament

Sacrotuberous ligament

Sciatic nerve

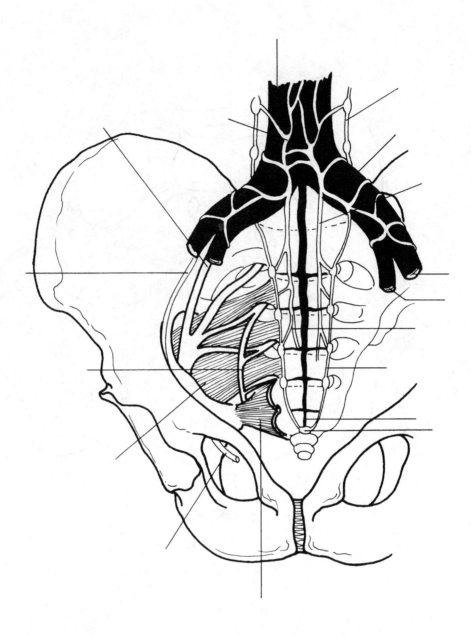

Abdominal aorta

Aortic plexus

Coccygeus muscle

Common iliac artery

External iliac artery

Ganglion impar

Inferior hypogastric plexus

Internal iliac artery

Lumbar sympathetic trunk

Lumbosacral trunk

Median sacral artery

Obturator nerve

Pelvic sympathetic trunk

Piriformis muscle

Pudendal nerve

Superior hypogastric plexus

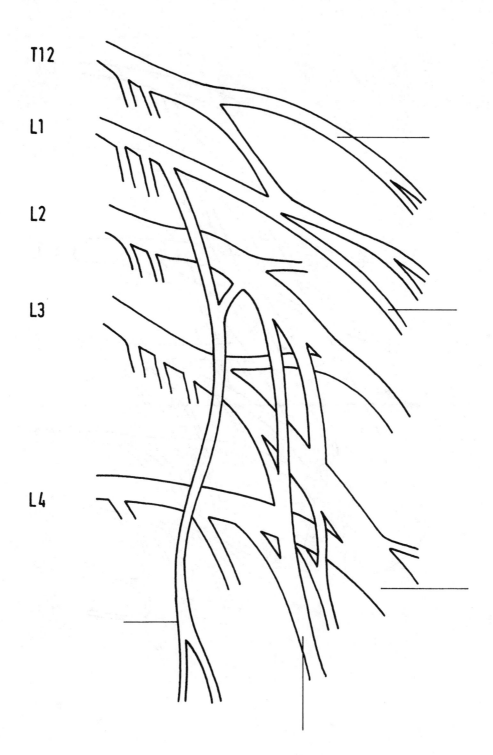

T12

L1

L2

L3

L4

Femoral nerve

Genitofemoral nerve

Ilioinguinal nerve

Obturator nerve

Subcostal nerve

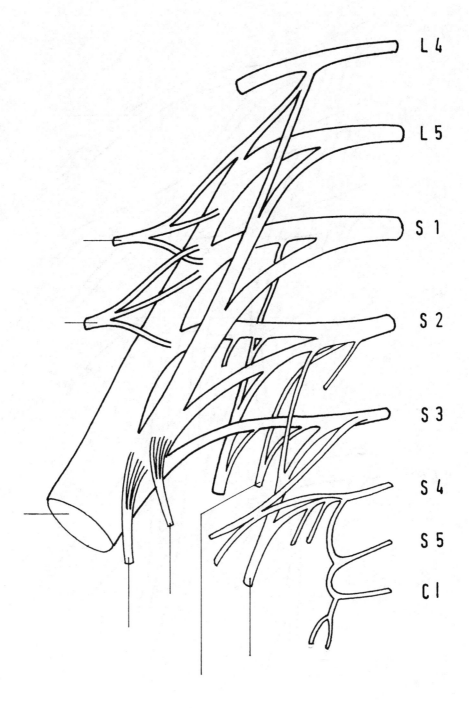

L 4

L 5

S 1

S 2

S 3

S 4

S 5

C I

Inferior gluteal nerve

Nerve to obturator internus

Nerve to quadratus femoris & inferior gemellus

Perforating cutaneous nerve

Pudendal nerve

Sciatic nerve composed of common peroneal & tibial components

Superior gluteal nerve

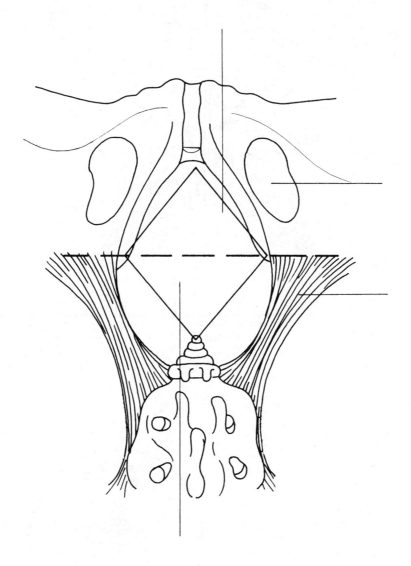

Anal triangle

Obturator foramen

Sacrotuberous ligament

Urogenital triangle

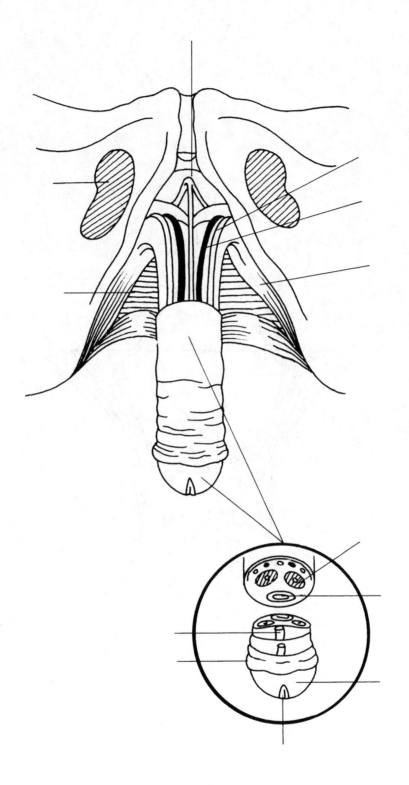

Corpora cavernosa

Corpus spongiosum

Deep dorsal vein

Dorsal artery

Dorsal nerve

External urethral meatus

Glans penis

Left crus of penis

Obturator membrane

Perineal membrane

Prepuce

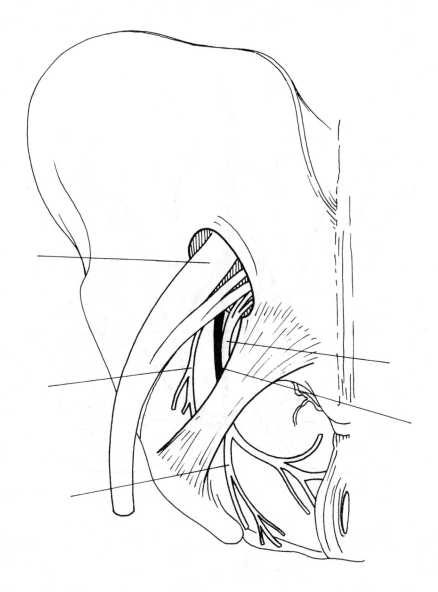

Internal pudendal artery

Lumbosacral trunk

Nerve to obturator internus

Pudendal nerve

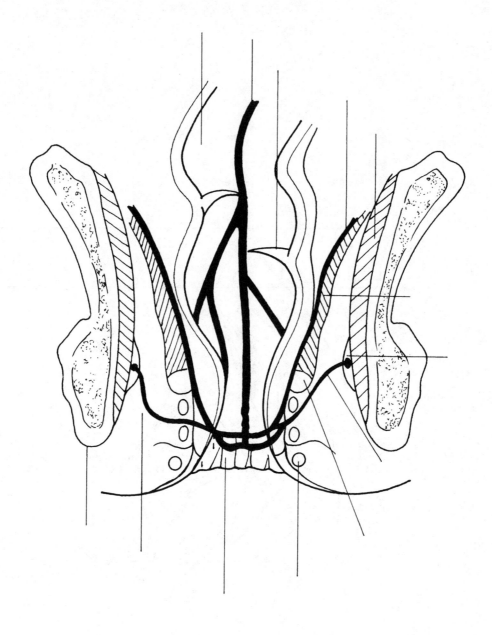

Anal valve

External anal sphincter

Inferior rectal vein

Ischiorectal fossa

Ischium

Levator ani

Middle rectal vein

Obturator internus

Puborectalis

Pudendal canal

Rectum

Superior rectal vein

Transverse fold of rectum

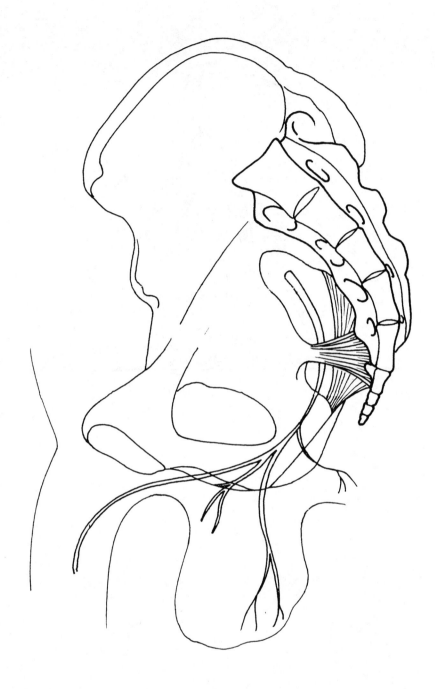

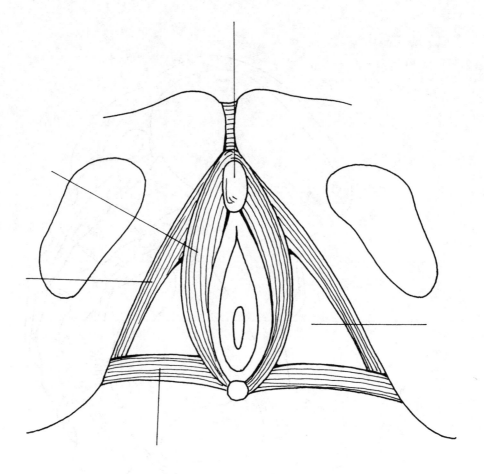

Bulbospongiosus muscle

Clitoris

Ischiocavernosus muscle

Perineal membrane

Transversus perinei superficialis
muscle

Section 6
LOWER LIMB

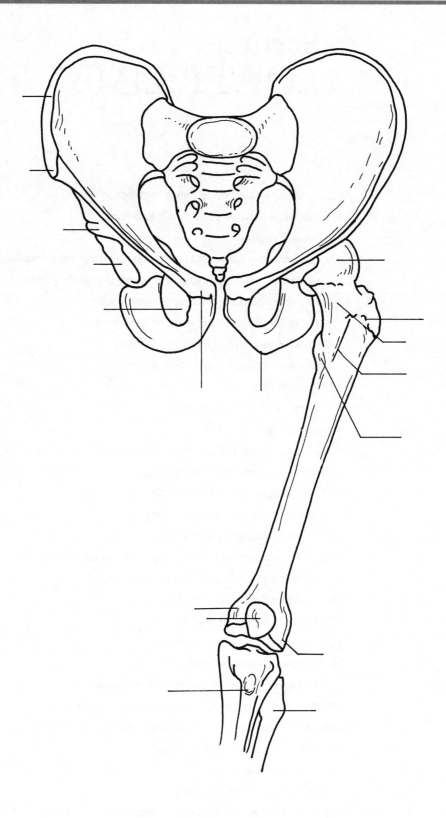

Acetabulum	Head of fibula	Neck of femur
Adductor tubercle	Iliac crest	Obturator foramen
Anterior inferior iliac spine	Intertrochanteric line	Patella
Anterior superior iliac spine	Ischial tuberosity	Pubis
Greater trochanter	Lateral condyle of femur	Tibial tuberosity
Head of femur	Lesser trochanter	

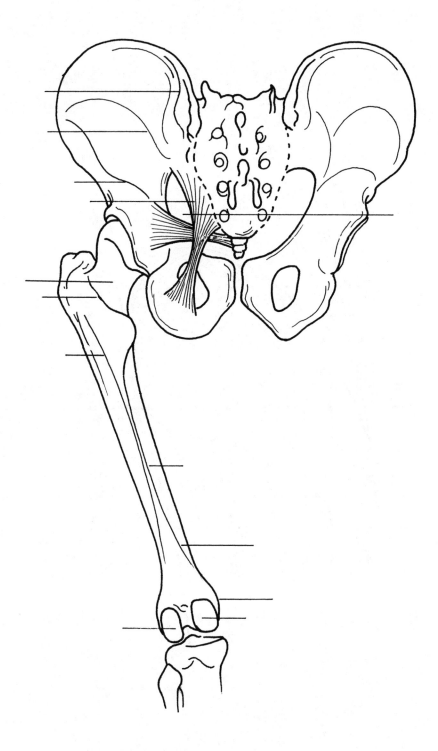

Adductor tubercle

Anterior gluteal line

Greater sciatic foramen

Inferior gluteal line

Intertrochanteric crest

Lateral and medial femoral
condyles

Linea aspera

Medial supracondylar line

Posterior gluteal line

Sacrotuberous ligament

Spiral line

Trochanteric fossa

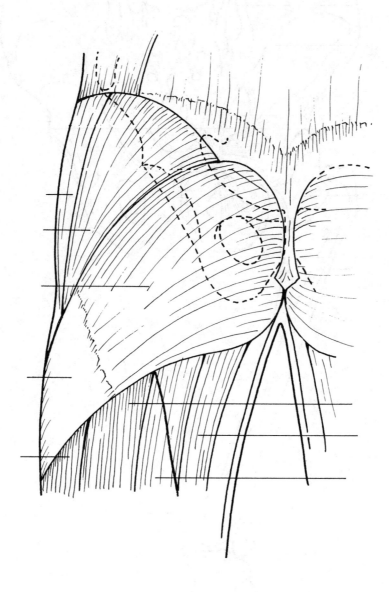

Gluteus maximus   Long head of biceps

Gluteus medius   Semimembranosus

Gracilis   Semitendinosus

Iliotibial tract   Tensor fasciae latae

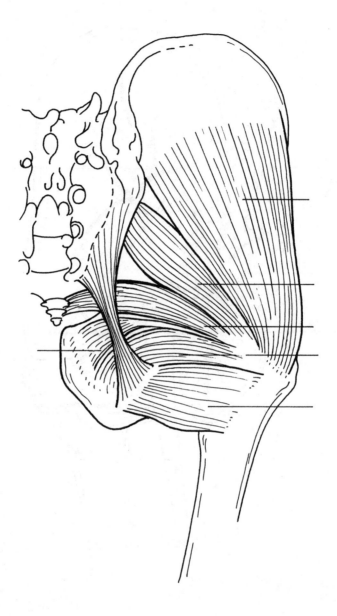

Gluteus minimus   Piriformis

Inferior gemellus   Quadratus femoris

Obturator internus   Superior gemellus

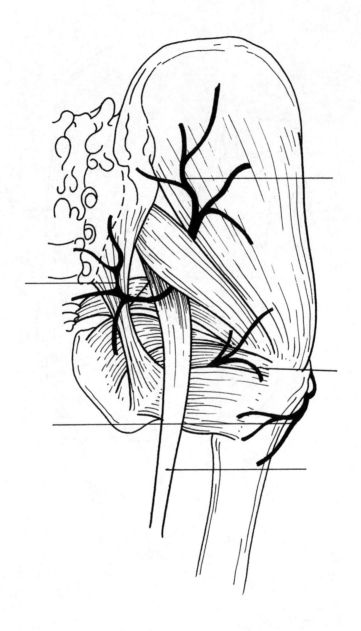

Inferior gluteal artery

Lateral circumflex femoral artery

Medial circumflex femoral artery

Sciatic nerve

Superior gluteal artery

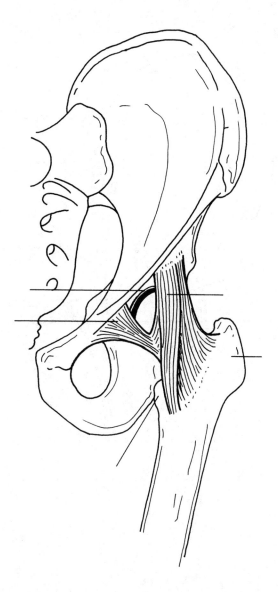

Acetabular labrum

Greater trochanter

Iliofemoral ligament

Lesser trochanter

Pubofemoral ligament

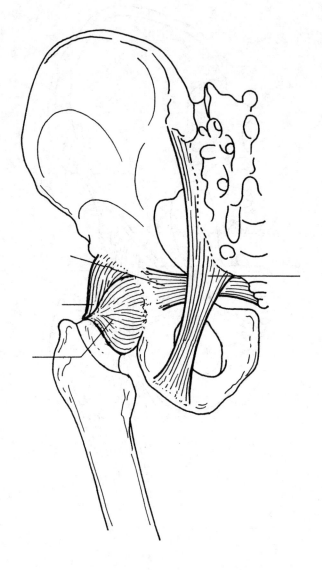

Iliofemoral ligament

Ischiofemoral ligament

Sacrospinous ligament

Sacrotuberous ligament

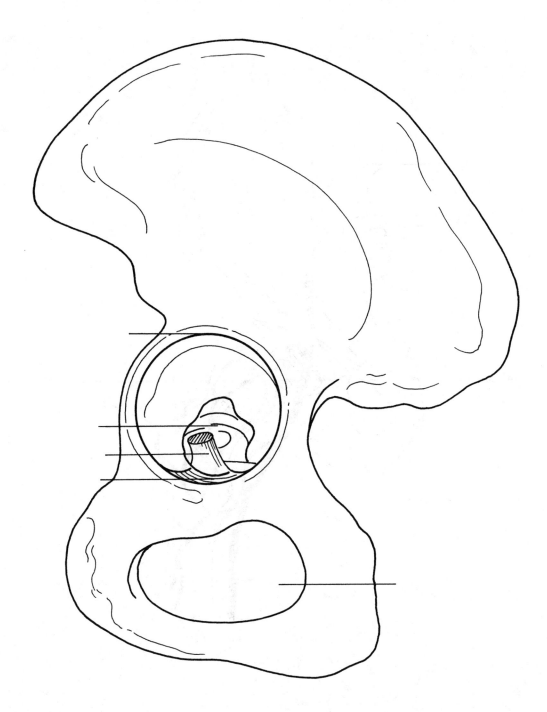

Fat pad of acetabulum

Ligament of head of femur

Obturator foramen

Rim of labrum

Transverse ligament

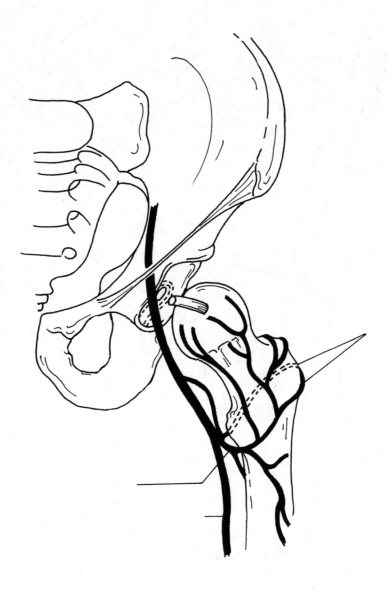

Circumflex femoral arteries

Femoral artery

Profunda femoris artery

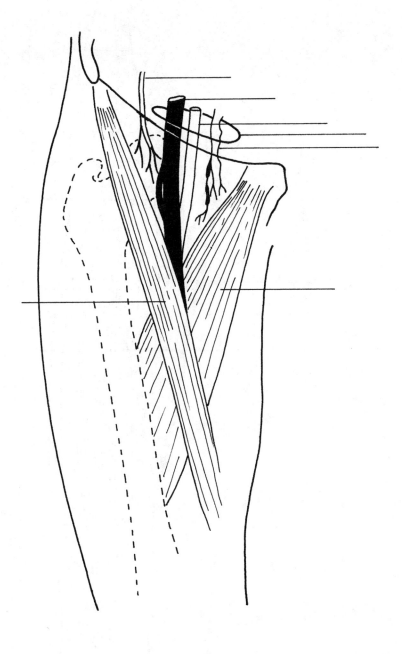

Adductor longus

Femoral artery

Femoral nerve

Femoral ring

Femoral vein

Lymphatics

Sartorius

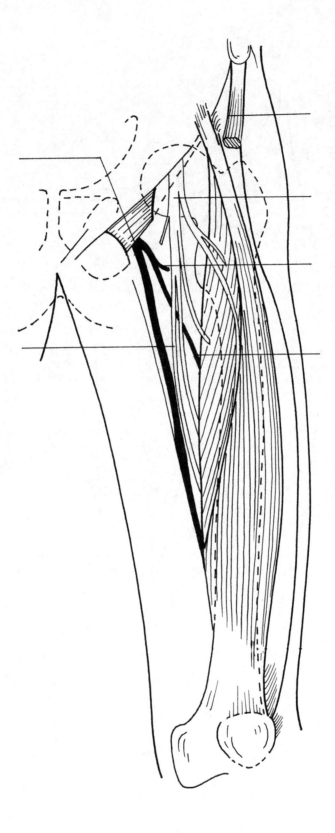

Cut end of sartorius   Lateral femoral circumflex artery

Femoral artery   Medial cutaneous nerve of thigh

Femoral nerve   Profunda femoris artery

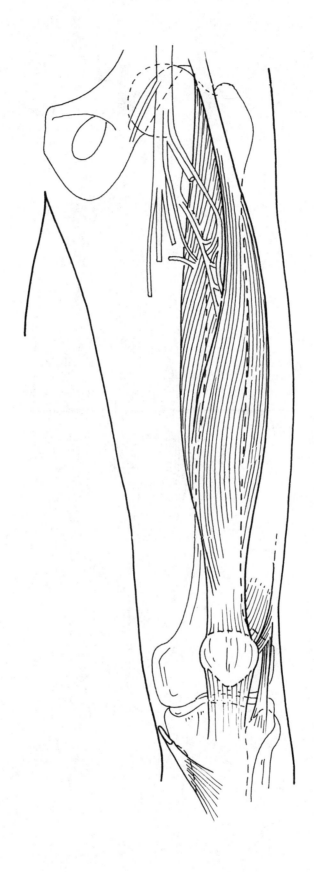

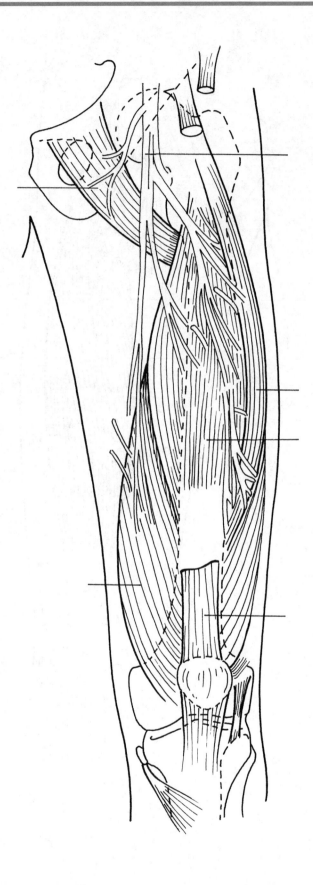

Femoral nerve	Vastus intermedius
Pectineus	Vastus lateralis
Rectus femoris (cut end)	Vastus medialis

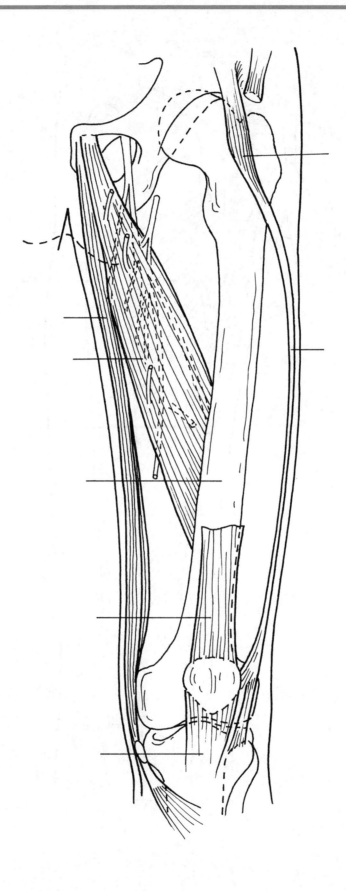

Adductor longus

Femur

Gracilis

Iliotibial tract

Ligamentum patellae

Rectus femoris (cut end)

Tensor fasciae latae

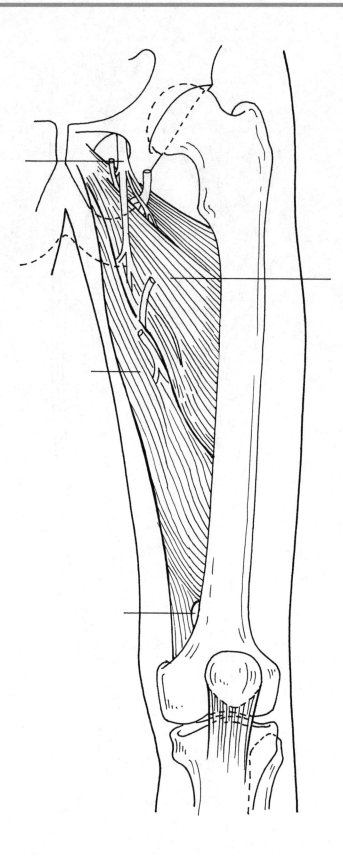

Adductor brevis

Adductor magnus

Obturator nerve

Opening in adductor magnus

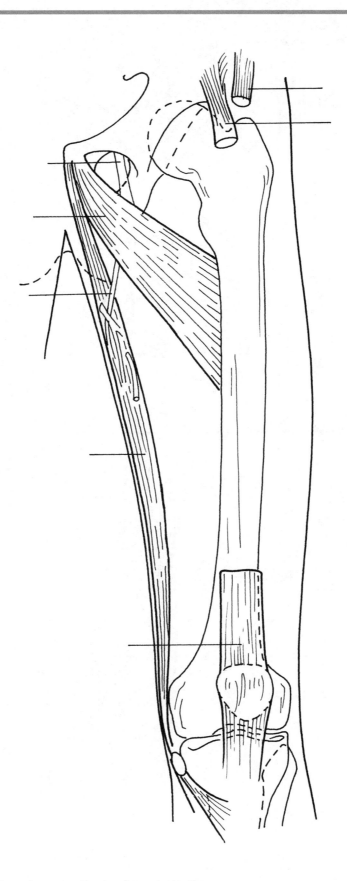

Branch of anterior division of obturator nerve

Gracilis

Obturator nerve

Pectineus

Rectus femoris (cut)

Sartorius (cut)

Tensor fasciae latae (cut)

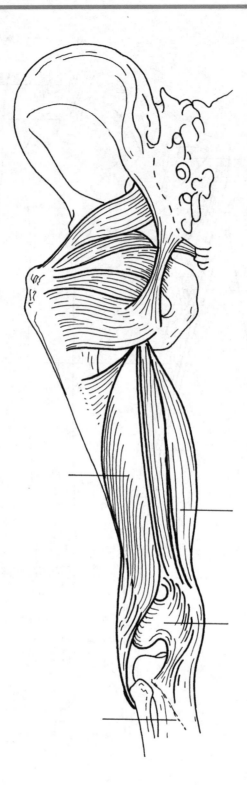

Biceps femoris

Posterior oblique ligament

Semimembranosus

Soleal line

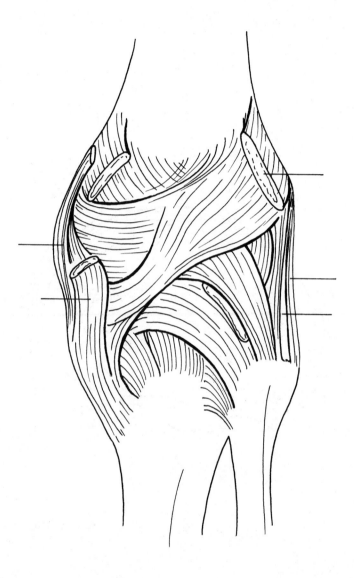

Fibular collateral ligament   Semimembranosus

Gap for tendon of popliteus   Tibial collateral ligament

Lateral head of gastrocnemius

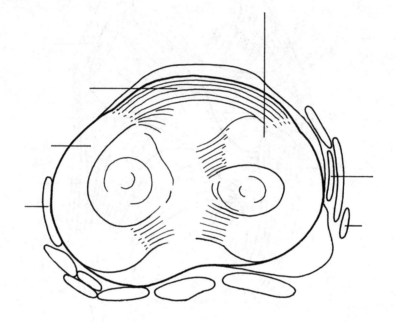

Fibular collateral ligament   Popliteus tendon

Lateral meniscus   Tibial collateral ligament

Medial meniscus   Transverse ligament

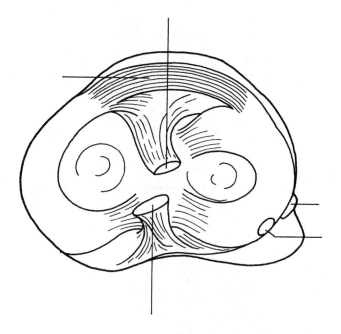

Anterior cruciate ligament

Lateral collateral ligament

Popliteus tendon

Posterior cruciate ligament

Transverse ligament

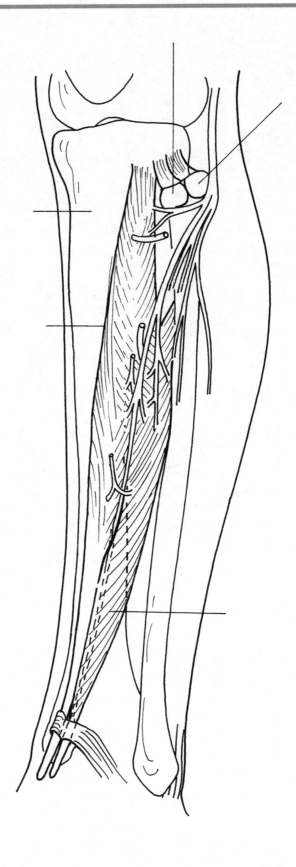

Extensor digitorum longus (cut)

Extensor hallucis longus

Peroneus longus (cut)

Tibia

Tibialis anterior

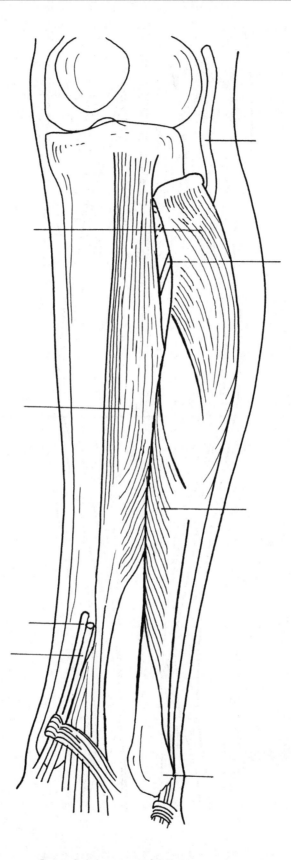

Common peroneal nerve

Extensor digitorum longus

Lateral malleolus

Peroneus brevis

Peroneus longus

Superficial peroneal nerve

Tendon of extensor hallucis longus

Tendon of tibialis anterior

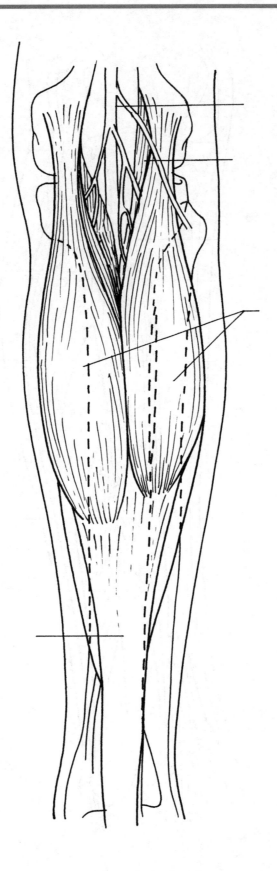

Lateral and medial heads of
gastrocnemius

Plantaris

Tendo calcaneus

Tibial nerve

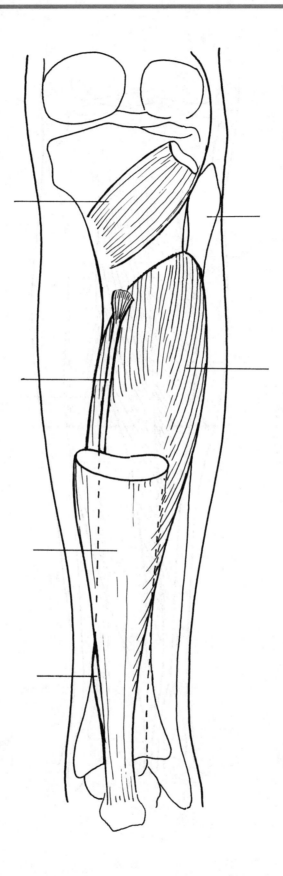

Head of fibula

Plantaris tendon

Popliteus (cut)

Soleus

Tendo calcaneus

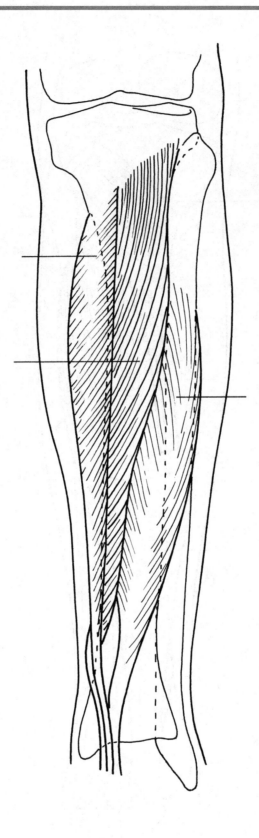

Flexor digitorum longus

Flexor hallucis longus

Tibialis posterior

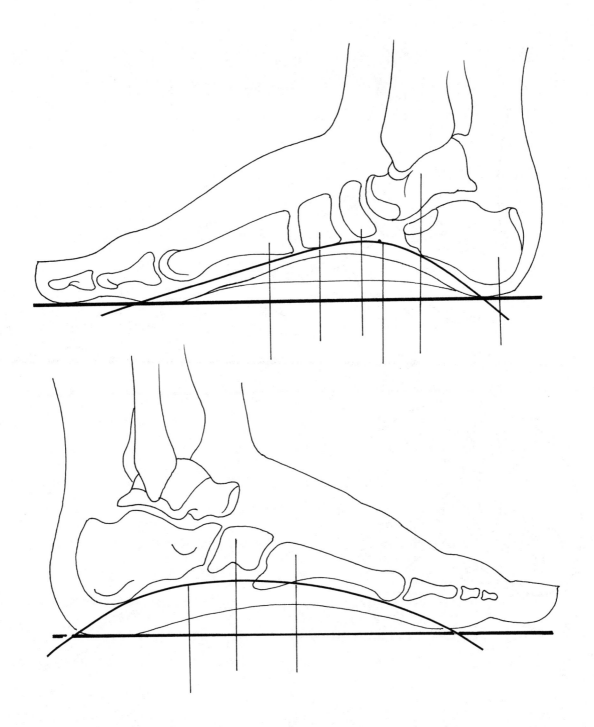

Calcaneus	Medial (1st) cuneiform bone	Metatarsal (5th) bone
Cuboid bone	Medial longitudinal arch	Navicular bone
Lateral longitudinal arch	Metatarsal (1st) bone	Talus

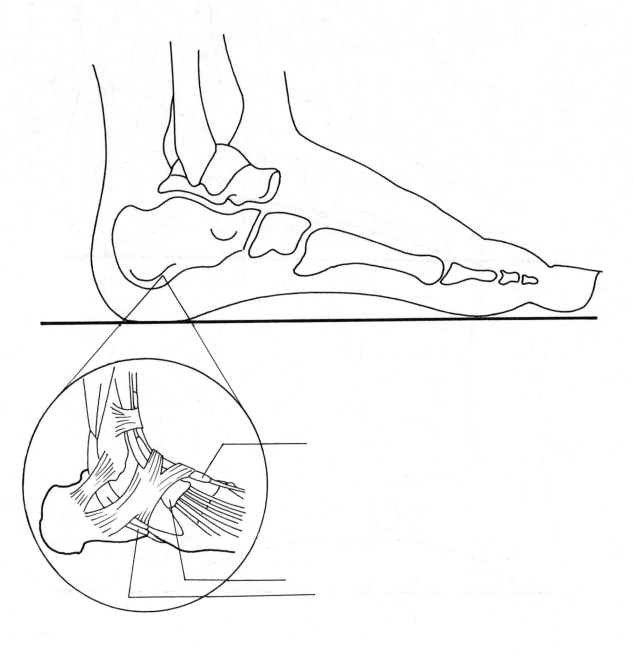

Synovial sheath of extensor
digitorum longus

Synovial sheath of extensor
hallucis longus

Synovial sheath of peroneus
longus

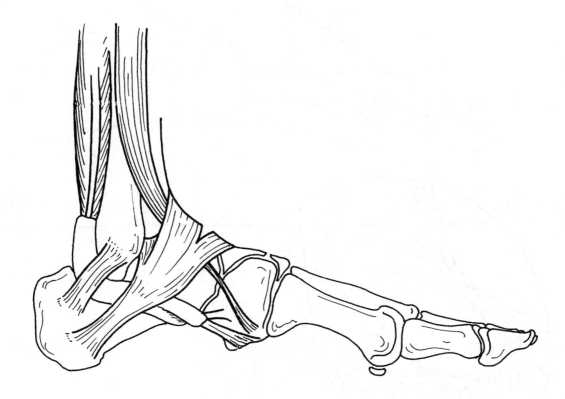

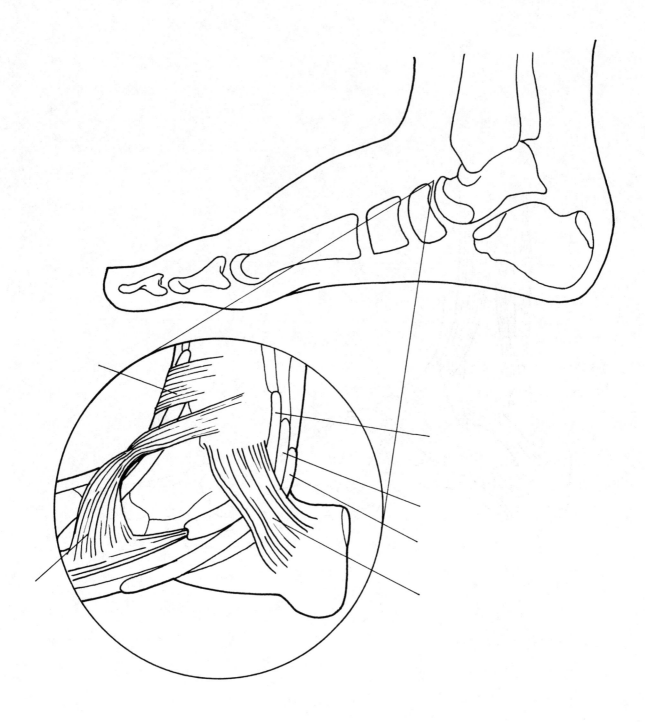

Flexor retinaculum

Inferior extensor retinaculum

Superior extensor retinaculum

Synovial sheath of flexor
digitorum longus

Synovial sheath of flexor hallucis
brevis

Synovial sheath of tibialis
posterior

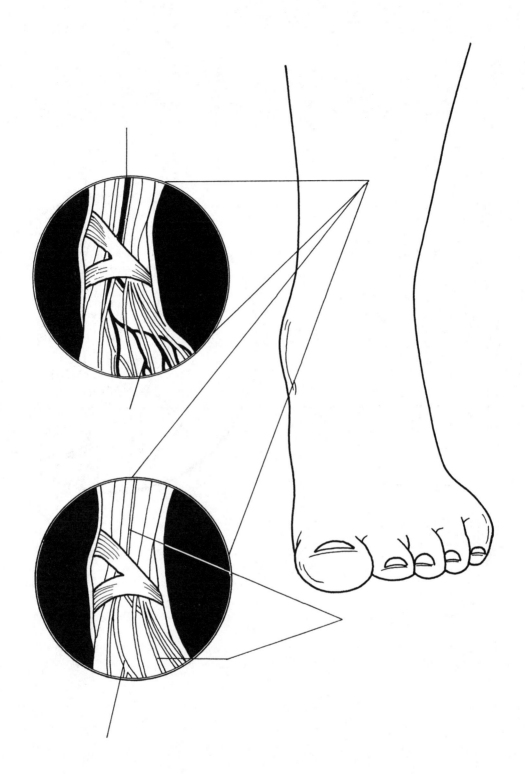

Anterior tibial artery

Deep peroneal nerve

Dorsal metatarsal artery

Superficial peroneal nerve

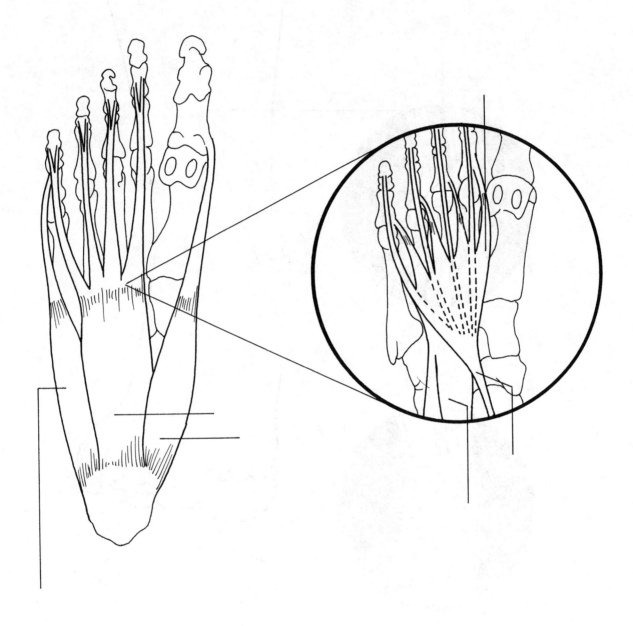

Abductor digiti minimi

Abductor hallucis

Flexor accessorius

Flexor digitorum brevis

Lumbricals

Tendon of flexor digitorum longus

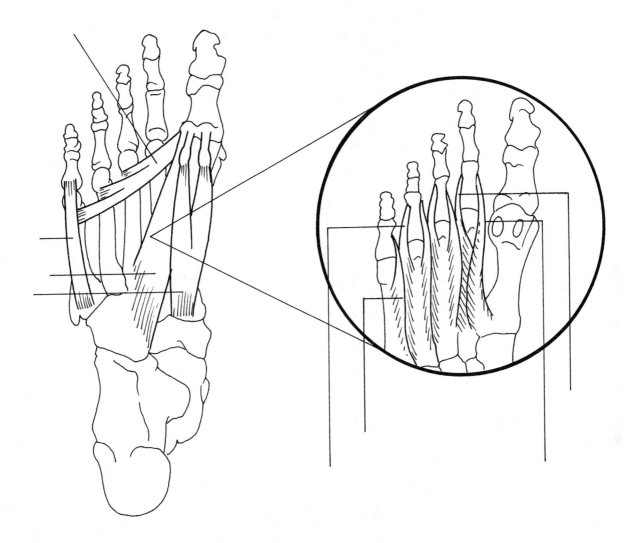

Adductor hallucis (oblique head)

Adductor hallucis (transverse head)

First dorsal interosseus

First plantar interosseus

Flexor digiti minimi brevis

Flexor hallucis brevis

Fourth dorsal interosseus

Third plantar interosseus

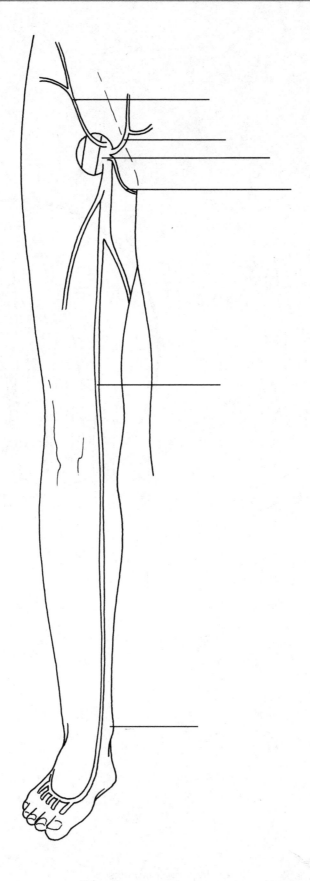

Femoral vein

Great saphenous vein

Medial malleolus

Superficial epigastric vein

Superficial external iliac vein

Superficial external pudendal vein